# Contesting Psychiatry

Sociologists have written much about power in relation to psychiatry and mental health services. Until now, however, there has been little research on resistance to this power, whether in the form of individual crusades or the collective efforts of social movements. As a result, a central thread in the social constitution of the mental health system has been overlooked.

*Contesting Psychiatry* explores the history of resistance to psychiatry in the UK between 1950 and 2000, and more particularly, the history of the social movements which have mounted this resistance, calling psychiatry into question. Key features include:

- an account of the key social movements and organisations which have contested psychiatry over the last fifty years
- an exploration of theories and conceptions of social movements as they apply in the health domain
- a theorisation of resistance to psychiatry which might apply to other national contexts and to social movement formation and protest in other medical arenas.

Original and provocative in its approach, *Contesting Psychiatry* offers a new sociological perspective on psychiatry. It is essential reading for students and academics alike and a unique contribution to the sociological understanding of psychiatry and medicine.

**Nick Crossley** is a Professor of Sociology at the University of Manchester, UK. His previous books include: *Making Sense of Social Movements* (2002, OUP), *The Politics of Subjectivity* (1994, Ashgate), *Intersubjectivity* (1996, Sage), *The Social Body* (2001, Sage) and *Key Concepts in Critical Social Theory* (2004, Sage).

**Critical Studies in Health and Society**
Series Editors
Simon J. Williams & Gillian Bendelow

This major new international book series takes a critical look at health in a rapidly changing social world. The series includes theoretically sophisticated and empirically informed contributions on cutting-edge issues from leading figures within the sociology of health and allied disciplines and domains. Current authors/titles include the following:

**New Social Movements and Mental Health**
*Nick Crossley*

**Men, Masculinities and Health**
*Alan Dolan*

**Medical Understandings of Lifestyles**
*Gary Easthope and Emily Hansen*

**Medical Sociology and Old Age**
Towards a sociology of health in later life
*Paul Higgs and Ian Rees Jones*

**Violence against Health Professionals**
*Jonathan Gabe*

**New Health Technologies and the Lifeworld**
*Sonja Olin Lauritzen, Lars-Christer Hydén and*
*Fredrik Svenaeus*

**Emotional Labour and Health Care**
*Catherine Theodosphius*

Written in a lively, accessible and engaging style, with many thought-provoking insights, the series will cater to a truly interdisciplinary audience of researchers, professionals, practitioners and policy makers with an interest in health and social change.

Those interested in submitting proposals for single or co-authored, edited or co-edited volumes should contact the series editors Simon Williams (s.j.williams@ warwick.ac.uk) and Gillian Bendelow (g.a.bendelow@sussex.ac.uk)

# Contesting Psychiatry
## Social movements in mental health

Nick Crossley

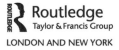
Routledge
Taylor & Francis Group

LONDON AND NEW YORK

First published 2006
by Routledge
2 Park Square, Milton Park, Abingdon, Oxon OX14 4RN

Simultaneously published in the USA and Canada
by Routledge
711 Third Ave, New York, NY 10017

*Routledge is an imprint of the Taylor & Francis Group*

Transferred to Digital Printing 2006

Typeset in Sabon by
Newgen Imaging Systems (P) Ltd, Chennai, India

*British Library Cataloguing in Publication Data*
A catalogue record for this book is available
from the British Library

*Library of Congress Cataloging in Publication Data*
Crossley, Nick, 1968–
    Contesting psychiatry : social movements in mental health /
Nick Crossley.
        p. ; cm. – (Critical studies in health and society)
    Includes bibliographical references and index.
    1. Antipsychiatry–Social aspects–Great Britain–History.
2. Mental health services–Great Britain–History. 3. Social
psychiatry–Great Britain–History. 4. Social movements–Great
Britain–History. I. Title. II. Series.
    [DNLM: 1. Psychiatry–history–Great Britain. 2. History,
20th Century–Great Britain. 3. Mental Health
Services–history–Great Britain. 4. Patient Rights–history–Great
Britain. 5. Public Opinion–Great Britain. 6. Social
Change–history–Great Britain. 7. Social Control
Policies–history–Great Britain. WM 11 FA1 C951c 2006]
    RC437.5.C77 2006
    362.2′0941–dc22                                    2005018080

ISBN10: 0–415–35416–1 (hbk)
ISBN10: 0–415–35417–X (pbk)

ISBN13: 9–78–0–415–35416–5 (hbk)
ISBN13: 9–78–0–415–35417–2 (pbk)

This book is dedicated to Jakey A.J. Crossley (11 months old), who is too young to have read the manuscript but who did chew over one or two of the chapters.

# Contents

# Illustrations

## Figures

## Tables

# Acknowledgements

The research upon which this book is based was funded in large part by a grant from the Economic and Social Research Council (ref. 00222187). Many thanks to them for their support. The writing up was completed during a teaching buyout funded partly by Manchester University's Centre for Research in Socio-Cultural Change (CRESC), to which I belong, and partly by the Sociology discipline area, to which I also belong. Again, thanks to both. I promise I'll get on with what I said I was going to do now!

I began this project whilst working at the Centre for Psychotherapeutic Studies in the Department of Psychiatry at the University of Sheffield. I finished it whilst working in what was the Department of Sociology at the University of Manchester (what is now the sociology 'discipline area'). Each of these locations has had a large impact upon the project and I am very grateful to colleagues at both for their support and input. It's been challenging and fun, in no small part because of you.

Thanks as ever go to Michele, who has kept me on my toes, intellectually and every other way, throughout, and to little Jakey who always reminds me that there is a life beyond the academic world – a wonderful life in fact.

Finally, thank you to the activists who allowed me to interview them and, in many cases, fed me a diet of documents relating to their groups, movements and causes. I have a great deal of respect for all of the people I interviewed and though you can't all 'win', whatever that entails, I wish you all well in your struggle. Whatever side of the fence one sits on, it is pretty obvious that much needs to be done to improve mental health services in the United Kingdom and it is due to people like you that it just might be.

# Introduction
## Researching resistance

This book is about the 'field of contention' that grew up around psychiatry and mental health services in Britain in the second half of the twentieth century. That is to say, it is about the interactions of competing and conflicting agents who sought to transform both conceptions and practices within the mental health system and the treatment of the 'mentally ill' in wider society. I focus not only upon groups who have opposed conventional psychiatry, pioneering their own alternatives, but also upon groups who have countered this opposition, calling upon mainstream psychiatry to ignore its liberal and radical critics and to stick to its 'proper role'.

The project upon which the book is based first began to take shape in the mid-1990s. I was working in a 'Centre for Psychotherapeutic Studies', in a Department of Psychiatry, teaching aspects of the sociology and philosophy of mental health to postgraduate students. I had decided to base a research project around this teaching interest and the imbalance in the curriculum pointed me in a very obvious direction. It seemed that almost every perspective in sociology had something to say about psychiatry and in most cases what they had to say centred upon issues of power and control. Much less, in fact scarcely anything at all, was written about resistance to this power and control. Foucauldian work was very much in the ascendancy in British sociology at the time and the early British Foucauldians, many of whom had cut their empirical teeth on 'psy' issues, were quite critical of what they took to be simplistic 'social control' approaches to the sociology of psychiatry (e.g. Miller 1986). However, 'power' was still central to their understanding of 'the psy-complex' (Miller and Rose 1986, Rose 1985, 1989), as it had been to Foucault (1965, 1987) and to French sociologists inspired by him (Castel 1988). Beyond the Foucauldians, there were prominent contributions from Marxist writers (Scull 1984, 1993), interactionists (Goffman 1961, 1971, Lemert 1951, Scheff 1984), feminists (Busfield 1996, Showalter 1987, Ussher 1991) and theorists of race and ethnicity (Fernando 1991, Littlewood and Lipsedge 1989, Sashidharan 1986), all of whom pointed in some way to the power and controlling function of psychiatry. Even less politically charged and more general accounts, such as we find in Parsons' (1951) reflections upon 'the sick role', essentially describe and name a process of social control. As noted earlier, however, what was much less evident was any attention to resistance to this power and control. Many sociologists themselves opposed and in their own way resisted psychiatric power and control but this and other forms of resistance were seldom made thematic as a topic of analysis. Resistance, so it seemed, was a blind spot. And its absence from the analytic spotlight, to my mind, generated a very one-sided picture of the mental health field.

The Foucauldians, admittedly, had a concept of resistance but it was poorly developed and never seemed to find its way into their otherwise impressive empirical accounts (although, more recently, see Cresswell forthcoming). Goffman (1961) had ventured a little further, offering a typology of ways in which inmates accommodate to life in large mental hospitals, which included forms of resistance. But this typology didn't 'do' very much except indicate that some inmates do sometimes resist in a variety of ways. Sedgwick (1982) was much more directly interested in resistance but his primary concern was to challenge fashionable streams of anti-psychiatric thought in a head-on political–philosophical contest, rather than exploring the emergence and context of these ideas in a sociological fashion. In a roundabout way, the historian, Roy Porter (1987b), in a study that explores selected stories of relatively well-known 'mad persons', had the most to say about resistance. Many of his 'stories of the insane' were, at least in part, stories of resistance. But resistance was not thematic in his analysis and was not analytically dissected. It seemed, therefore, that I had found an area in need of analysis. I was going to investigate resistance to psychiatry.

My original inclination was to approach resistance at an individual level, focusing upon small gestures, such as omitting to take pills. I hoped to work observationally and in 'real time'. Perhaps I would observe on a ward? This quickly proved a dead end for both methodological and pragmatic reasons. Much individual level protest, insofar as one can tell, is conducted in secret or at least beyond the reach of the psychiatric gaze. It is conducted in private spaces where it is not amenable to observation and those who do it keep it private because they do not want to be identified. In addition, when resistance is more overt (e.g. a patient absconds) it happens unannounced and, to all intents and purposes, out of the blue. This makes observation and 'real-time' analysis very difficult. On top of this, the more I examined and thought about isolated acts of resistance, the more slippery their meaning became and the less sure I was that they could be described as acts of resistance. Omitting to take medicine, throwing it down the toilet or absconding can be motivated by a variety of factors: for example, forgetfulness, distraction, apathy, despondency, fear etc., not just opposition to psychiatry. In the medical sense of 'treatment resistance' these diverse motivations are of little consequence since anything that hinders treatment, for whatever reason, is regarded as resistance. Likewise psychoanalysis is inclined to read oppositional intent into a variety of seemingly innocent motivations. Sociology, however, must be more discriminating with respect to meaning. Are patients who forget to take their medication really resisting? Even absconding cannot unproblematically be deemed 'resistance', at least if motivated by an impulse of fear and an opportunity to run. Running from what one fears is not exactly resisting it. And neither is omitting or avoiding what is unpleasant. At least these are not examples of resistance with a capital 'R'.

Resistance, I began to think, implies a project of resistance which, even if it begins life in the form of vague, spontaneous and pre-reflective gestures and impulses, at some point becomes thematic and reflective, linking up to 'vocabularies of motive' (Mills 1967) which formulate it as resistance. Resistance is 'theorised' by those who engage in it. And these theories, in turn, steer and sustain it. The problem with individual and isolated acts of resistance, it became clear, was that I could not link them to reflexive projects of resistance which would constitute them as acts of resistance. And without reflexive projects of resistance I could not be clear that what I was looking at were acts of resistance at all.

One way out of this problem might have been to interview patients who engage in such acts in order to ascertain whether they define their acts in terms of resistance projects. However, this is easier said than done. On the one hand, as noted earlier, identifying patients who engage in these activities is difficult because the acts are often invisible. On the other, though my (always sympathetic) psychiatric colleagues would have supported and aided such a project wholeheartedly, medical ethics committees, who act as gatekeepers in such research, often prove less amenable. I felt that, methodologically, the open-ended and exploratory nature of an investigation of this kind would not appeal to their narrow and relatively conservative view of good research design (generally based on hypothetico-deductive and double-blind models). More importantly still, however, I had doubts about the methodology myself. Would interviews really give me access to what I was after in this situation? Wasn't there a risk that my results would turn out to be an artefact of my project; that I would put interviewees in a situation where they felt obliged to concoct stories of resistance for my benefit, or at least to thematise, reflect upon and make sense of behaviours that they would not ordinarily have given much thought or meaning to? Would I be turning what might otherwise, for my interviewees, be mundane and largely insignificant molehills into mountains of sociological research? This is always a danger in interview research, of course, including the research that I did eventually go on to do, but it seemed particularly acute in this context.

For these reasons it began to dawn upon me that publicly organised forms of resistance, which were the main source of my sense that there was resistance in the first place, might make a better focus for a sociological study. In public forms of resistance, agents freely identify themselves as 'opposed to psychiatry' or indeed, in favour of it. They register their views in documents which an interested social scientist can access and analyse. They have an explicit project of resistance and they spell it out in manifestos, magazines, books and meetings. There is, for this reason, less ambiguity at the level of meaning with respect to their acts of resistance. Furthermore, there are 'naturally occurring' data which are free of the potential contamination of sociological prompts. Public forms of resistance generally generate a paper trail which the sociologist can pick up and analyse.

The more I looked at instances of resistance and resisting individuals, defined in this way, the more I found them to be connected to collectives of various sorts. Although most individuals are capable of saying 'no' and refusing to comply and although there are many individual biographical trajectories into resistance, the maturing of individual sentiments and inclinations into projects of resistance is very often a collective phenomenon. Projects of resistance and the components they involve (e.g. identities, narratives, protest activities, vocabularies of motive) are much easier to generate and sustain collectively. Ideas develop and flourish in dialogue and agents can confirm for one another the 'reality' of what they are doing and opposing. The maintenance of even mundane and uncontroversial definitions of reality, as Berger and Luckmann (1979) note, often requires confirmation and complicity from others. This is all the more so when the definition in question runs contrary to and is critical of that proffered by symbolically and materially powerful agents. Moreover, group life generates an *esprit de corps* which binds members into their collective project (Blumer 1969) and networks of support which raise morale and keep the project afloat when downturns threaten. Resources can be pooled and labour shared. And groups and networks recruit, intentionally and unintentionally, thereby generating pathways into resistance which others may follow and may find easier to tread than the self-made path of the pioneer.

The importance of the collective dimension led me to the literature on the sociology of protest, social movements and what Tilly (1978) and Tarrow (1998) call 'contentious politics' (see Crossley 2002a). Working through this literature, I elected to map collective resistance of contentious politics in the mental health domain in terms of three key elements: (1) social movements, (2) social movement organisations (SMOs) and (3) fields of contention. These concepts are explained in detail in Chapter 1. Suffice it to say for now that I define social movements, very loosely, as emergent discourses within a society or subsection of society which constitute or connect to a political demand. I define SMOs, following Zald and McCarthy (1994), as specific organisations, groups, networks or projects which represent, service, cultivate and act upon that demand in pursuit of its goal, sometimes in competition or conflict with one another. I define a field of contention as the dynamic, always-in-process social and cultural structure generated by way of the interactions and relationships both between SMOs and between SMOs and a range of further relevant players who are implicated in the problems or issues identified in social movement discourses. The other relevant players referred to here include funding bodies that SMOs might apply to, agents of social control who seek to restrict and regulate their activity, government departments, and pools of 'adherents' and 'constituents' (see Chapter 1).

There may be more than one movement represented in any field of contention, as, indeed, there are often many competing SMOs seeking to represent a single movement. The field of psychiatric contention is a good example of this. Between 1950 and 2000, the period I cover in this study, it has been populated by at least five distinct social movements, all of which are discussed in this book and most of which have been represented by more than one SMO at any point of time:

1   a mental hygiene movement;
2   a civil rights movement;
3   an anti-psychiatry movement;
4   a movement which began as a 'patients'' movement but later renamed itself a 'user' or 'survivor' movement, and then later, for some at least, became a 'mad' movement and
5   a movement which has no obvious label but which tends to represent the interests of the families of 'the mentally ill', which is critical of liberalism and radicalism in psychiatry, calling for quicker diagnosis and treatment, and which therefore tends to be critical of and criticised by activists and SMOs in movements 2, 3 and 4: an anti-anti-psychiatry movement.

The mental hygiene movement slightly predates the others and had more or less faded out before the patient and anti-anti-psychiatry movements had emerged. It coexisted, not altogether peacefully, with the civil rights and anti-psychiatry movements, however. And the others have coexisted with one another, again not always peacefully, in more recent times. This interplay of different movements and their SMOs, within a single field of contention which they collectively constitute, is one of the key foci of this study.

Posing the question of resistance in terms of movements, SMOs and fields, it will now be obvious, raises a historical aspect. Fields are, as noted, always 'in process'. Movements and SMOs come and go within them and change their patterns of alliance and relationships, as indeed do funding bodies and government departments. The question therefore arises of where specific movements and SMOs come from. Why do they emerge where they do, when they do, in the way that they do? These are key questions for this study. In addition, however, I have also been interested in questions of stability and reproduction; how do movements and SMOs manage to survive and maintain their identity and stability over time, given their own processual nature and the often changing dynamics of the field in which they are involved?

Sociological theories are useful in answering these questions and I have situated my analysis within a strong theoretical framework, which is outlined in Chapter 1. Equally important, however, is the historical narrative of the field, its movements and their SMOs. To understand a field and its 'parts' (i.e. movements, SMOs and activists) we need to understand its 'story'; that is, how events, episodes, SMOs etc. unfold and connect across time. Moreover, we need to make space for the events and contingencies that often assume a central place in these stories. Sociologists are often reluctant to focus on 'story' in this way, partly because of concerns that analysis might collapse into 'mere description' and partly because of the tacit nomothetic bias of the discipline, which makes contingencies and particularities difficult to engage with. However, we need to move beyond this position. First, we must recognise that narratives and descriptions always already embody a considerable amount of analytic work. Second, we need to recognise that narratives in particular access and analyse a central aspect of social reality which tends to elude other research approaches: its temporal flow and processual nature. Third, as Andrew Abbott (2001) has argued, sociological explanation cannot begin to get off the ground without strong descriptions and narratives which pull together the available data. I am not proposing to abandon all conventional sociological models and forms of analysis in favour of 'the story'. Clearly both are important and the line between them can become very blurred. But 'the story' is important in this study, and I want to prepare the reader for that and briefly explain myself.

## Questions of method

Mention of 'the story' raises further questions: how have I pieced it together and where has my data come from? My initial inclination was to access the field by way of an analysis of the archives of written material produced by the relevant SMOs. In the event, however, following a successful application for a small grant to the *Economic and Social Research Council* (ESRC),[1] I was able to supplement my archive analysis with a series of oral history interviews with 'key players' from the various groups I was identifying; that is to say, activists who had been involved in setting up groups, who had been involved in a number of groups and/or had achieved a high profile in the field. Totally, 35 key players were interviewed. Moreover, as no formal archive existed for most of the SMOs I was becoming interested in, archive compilation became as much a part of my project as archive analysis, and this tended to run alongside the interview process. In the course of my interviews I asked interviewees if they had kept any of the documentation of the various groups and campaigns they had been involved in. Some had kept a great deal, including manifestos, newssheets and minutes of meetings, and most were willing to allow me to make copies of what they had. In this way I was able to build an archive consisting of over 50 A4 document wallets of materials, which filled 3 large storage boxes.

Interviewees were selected, in part, by way of a snowball sample. I asked each of my interviewees who the key players in the field were and whether they had contact details for these people. I then chased up these people and repeated the process until no new names came up. In addition, I selected interviewees from the archive, looking out for names which tended to crop up repeatedly. When I had identified a person in this way I contacted them by whatever channels were open to me and requested an interview. I didn't interview everybody who was on my wish list. Some had died. Others did not respond to my letters or phone messages. I was, however, able to interview many of the key players from UK mental health politics, particularly from the 1980s and 1990s.

The interviews, which all lasted between 30 minutes and 2 hours (except for two email interviews), were open ended but focused primarily upon individual histories of activism and the histories of specific SMOs. They are cited anonymously in the text with an interview number and, where relevant, a brief description of the interviewee (e.g. 'psychiatrist'). Interview numbers reflect the order of first appearance of the interviews in the body of my text, such that the first interview I use is cited as 'Interview 1' throughout the study, the second as 'Interview 2' etc. (not all interviews are cited in the study).[2] It has sometimes proved difficult to reconcile the imperative of anonymity with the broader nature of my project. The history I am recounting is replete with 'stars' of various kinds, some of whom I have had to name as actors in the drama, since doing otherwise would render my account absurd – like a history of the kings and queens of England which omitted their names. Activists, almost by definition, generate publicity for their causes and, by default, for themselves. Moreover, they write, sometimes prolifically, attaching their own names to what they write. It has been difficult sometimes to discuss a named individual and their writing and then cite interview material with them whilst keeping them anonymous. I hope, however, that I have succeeded.

I approached the analysis of interview transcripts and archive documents in three ways. Some, which spoke directly of the history I was attempting to trace, I treated as 'witness statements'. I was aware, of course, that witness statements are often partial, on account of the location and interests of the witness. They don't see everything and neither do they say everything that they did see. They are selective and they may have an investment in telling the story one way rather than another. I was seldom in a situation where I had only one account of major events to draw upon, however, and was thus able, through a process of cross-checking and corroboration, to piece together an account which was agreed upon by a number of independent sources. Other documents didn't so much report upon the history I was tracing as belong to it. They were minutes of meetings, newssheets, posters and flyers; speech acts produced in the heat of a moment but now frozen in time on a photocopied sheet before me. These documents too recorded and reported on events, and I was able to use them as direct evidence, drawing information from them about events, relationships, issues etc. Moreover, both these and my witness statements served the purpose of directing me to further possible sources of evidence. Some, for example, refer to media articles, debates in Parliament or published books. Finally, in relation to all documents and interview transcripts, I adopted a stance that was more 'phenomenological' in nature. I was interested to see how different writers and speakers 'constructed' their domain; how issues were framed, what language was used and what assumptions made; what was taken for granted and what thematised; who was referenced and referred to and what this might say about the referee, referent and their relationship. Inspired by Mead (1967) and Merleau-Ponty (1962, 1965), I took these discourses to be a concrete embodiment of the thought processes of the agents who produced them, albeit an embodiment in need of interpretation and one which could not be taken at face value; an embodiment which better allowed me to understand how they made sense of their own situations. The documents and transcripts contained vocabularies of motive and plans of action. They betrayed the typifications and reasoning processes of those who expressed them. Moreover, and of historical interest, they could be seen to change over time. Typifications and schemas which dominate at one point in time drop out of favour and are replaced at another time, thereby indicating discursive shifts. Interestingly, they also sometimes served as 'fingerprints', allowing me to roughly date documents and identify (probable) links between groups and activists. Tracing the migration of particular terms and symbols across different groups and campaigns, for example, allowed me to hypothesise links between the groups and campaigns themselves, which I could then follow up with further probing.

The final aspect of my research involved a wider reading of secondary sources on the history of both psychiatry and wider UK society during the period I was examining. I wanted to understand the evolving context to which mental health politics belonged and which might have affected it in various ways. Sometimes, of course, these wider events are referred to within the archive. I did not need to read the wider history, for example, to appreciate that mental health services were being transformed in the 1980s by an acceleration of the shift towards community care. The groups I was examining all made reference to this and, for some, it was central. Sometimes, however, wider events which have an impact upon activism are either too immediate and obvious or too distant for them to notice, such that they only really become apparent to the sociologist with the benefit of hindsight. To capture these factors, however, it is necessary to read the wider histories alongside the primary materials I was using. And that is what I did.

## Empirical limits

Has this study referenced every relevant and important SMO active in the UK field of psychiatric contention during the latter half of the twentieth century? No. In the first instance, my study is primarily focused upon the national level and affords only passing consideration to international and local developments, and only then when they are relevant to understanding the national level. This is a limitation of the study but, in my defence, it is always necessary to set the limits somewhere.

Perhaps more problematically, the 'national level' is not always easy to define. National SMOs generally have local headquarters and in the case of small SMOs, they generally lack regional or local offices. Some claim to represent the nation but in effect, tend to operate locally. And some are better placed, because of their location, to pass themselves off as national when they are no more so than other SMOs which tend to be regarded as local. This blurs the distinction between local and national. I am aware, for example, that I have tended to treat London based groups as 'national' (where they claim to be) even in cases where I know that their active membership and range of activities are all based in London. This is not my bias as such. My own base is not London and I would not have afforded priority to London-based groups if they did not appear to enjoy priority and national standing. But they did. In addition, I probably did introduce my own local bias. I began the project when located in Sheffield and finished it at my current Manchester base. I must surely therefore also have taken the claims to 'national significance' of Sheffield and Manchester based SMOs more seriously than similar groups in other localities which are less well known to me. I am aware for example that I was not able to pursue important developments in both Nottingham and Bristol to the same extent as I was able to pursue equally important developments in my home town(s) because the latter were so much easier to access and return to. And of course there may be developments in other places that I did not hear about. There is an interesting geo-politics to fields of contention that could be studied here. I have not studied it but I am aware that I may have been influenced by it.

Another effect which may have influenced me concerns the tendency towards differentiation in fields of contention. Although it is not possible to talk in terms of simple linear patterns of development in fields, one relatively durable trend that I have noted is towards differentiation. Over time, a field becomes more populated with SMOs and this generates a tendency for greater specialisation amongst these SMOs. Where early SMOs claimed to represent 'mental patients' in general, for example, many recent SMOs are more specific and deal with a particular 'condition' (e.g. manic-depression) or even specific 'symptoms' (e.g. hearing voices or paranoia). Likewise, where the early SMOs tended to take on all relevant issues we now find SMOs devoted specifically to tackling particular problems, such as ECT or a specific mental health policy. Finally, where early SMOs committed themselves to pursuing their struggle across many domains (e.g. the media, the courts, parliament, the psychiatric system itself) we now find some groups who specialise in very specific interventions (e.g. they focus upon the media) – or who have differentiated internally, developing offices corresponding to these different areas of intervention. As the field has become more heavily populated and differentiated it has not been possible for me to pay as much attention to each individual SMO. This is justifiable in this particular case because my concern has been, throughout, with the field of contention as a whole, and as that field has become more populated and busy it has been necessary to step back a little further from it in order to keep the whole in focus. Inevitably, however, it means that my account of earlier groups is richer than my account of later groups.

The later groups perhaps also lose out slightly in the respect that the interview period of my study ended in the late 1990s, annoyingly just before a number of interesting new developments at the end of the century. I was fortunate to meet and interview one of the key innovators of this later period (Peter Shaughnessy) before his sad death. So I had some sense of these new developments in their embryonic stages. When they did happen, however, I had my eye off the ball. I was working on other things. And I therefore had to retrospectively re-engage with these very late (in terms of my 'period') developments, working from documentary sources alone, when the opportunity for this book arose. That is unfortunate.

Finally, as one is forced to be selective in any study, I have tended to focus upon SMOs which appear to form a particular common narrative thread in the field; SMOs who interact with one another, sometimes cooperating but also often competing or conflicting and also who tend to refer to one another in their literature. Doubtless there are other threads and there are certainly other SMOs. I believe that I have identified the central thread, at least as far as the contentious politics of psychiatry is involved, however. I have identified the SMOs who have been most central in attempting to change psychiatry and mental health provision or preventing others from implementing their changes. In this respect I believe that I am offering a pretty reliable map of the field of psychiatric contention between 1950 and 2000, not to mention a sociologically interesting and relevant account of its dynamics and transformations.

## Chapter plan

Chapters 1–3 are focused upon important aspects of background to the main body of the study. Chapter 1 discusses the key concepts outlined in this chapter: social movements, SMOs and fields of contention. Chapter 2 outlines my theoretical model for explaining the emergence of movements. And Chapter 3 follows this up with a 'potted history' of psychiatry and mental health services in the United Kingdom.

Chapter 4 opens the analysis proper. I focus primarily upon the 1950s but also look backwards to the 1930s and 1940s in an effort to account for the birth of the first important SMO of the post-1950s era: *The National Association for Mental Health* (NAMH). In the 1970s and 1980s, acting under the name MIND, this SMO was a radical campaign group pursuing a civil rights agenda. In the 1950s, however, they were key members of the international mental hygiene movement and acted very much as apologists for both mainstream psychiatry and government policy. This chapter explores some of the critiques that NAMH attempted to defend psychiatry from in the 1950s and does not seek to underplay the contention and controversy surrounding mental hospitals at this time. However, I regard this period, to some degree, as the calm before the storm and this is reflected in my account. Moreover, I try to draw out the conservativism and antagonism towards civil rights campaigns that characterised NAMH at this point in order that their later conversion to civil rights, discussed in Chapter 6, is properly appreciated.

The storm that followed this calm, in the form of the anti-psychiatry movement of the 1960s, is discussed in Chapter 5. The emergence of anti-psychiatry was a turning point in the field of contention which had long lasting implications and effects. I therefore devote a whole chapter to it.

Chapter 6 focuses upon three developments in the 1970s, each of which has at least some relationship to anti-psychiatry: the transformation of NAMH into MIND; the birth of the *National Schizophrenia Fellowship* (NSF – later renamed *Rethink*), an SMO who were critical of anti-psychiatry and the 'overly liberal' concerns of many psychiatrists; and the birth of *People Not Psychiatry*, an SMO which very much echoed and grew out of anti-psychiatry. Reflecting upon these three SMOs and their respective relations to anti-psychiatry and its SMOs affords us a sense of the field-like nature of mental health politics.

Chapter 7 focuses upon another development from the 1970s, also related to anti-psychiatry: the birth of the modern 'patients' movement, in the form of the *Mental Patients' Union* (MPU). The emergence of a patients' movement, like the birth of anti-psychiatry, was a major turning point in the history of the field. The MPU was the first in what became a succession of 'survivor' (as they were later called) SMOs.

Chapters 8 and 9 bring the story up to date. In Chapter 8 I trace the 'second waves' of both the anti-psychiatry and survivor movements, in the form of the *British Network for Alternatives to Psychiatry, Survivors Speak Out* and the *United Kingdom Advocacy Network* (UKAN), tracing the overlaps between these SMOs and with MIND. In Chapter 9 I trace the later history of the backlash against psychiatric radicalism and liberalism, in the form of SANE, exploring some of the battles between this SMO and its more liberal or radical contemporaries. And I consider the developments that were just taking off at the end of my period of study, in particular the formation of *Mad Pride* and *Reclaim Bedlam*.

Throughout all of these chapters I will be attempted to explore the processes and conditions involved in the birth of movements and SMOs, those involved in their survival and reproduction and also those involved in their decline. At the same time, however, I will maintain a constant focus upon the bigger picture of the field, trying to draw out the significance of relations and interactions between SMOs, both within and across movements. The field is a constant in this study, even if it changed beyond recognition through the period studied, and it is my primary referent.

## A note on language

Some of the SMOs and activists I have looked in this study have sought to challenge the language of psychiatry. Terms such as 'mental illness', 'the mentally ill', 'patients' etc. have been problematised and terms such as 'ex-patient', 'survivor', 'user' (of mental health services) and 'mental distress' have been developed and/or advocated. Indeed, 'madness' and 'lunacy' have been rejected as pejorative by one wave of reformers only to be rediscovered and reappropriated by at least some participants in a later wave. Particular camps at particular times usually agree with respect to linguistic practices but there is little agreement across camps and time, and even the homogeneity of camp-times tends to be short-lived and murky 'at the edges'.

I have tried to use language appropriately in this study, avoiding anachronism ('patients' were 'patients' even in radical circles in the 1970s) and trying to avoid putting inappropriate language in the mouths of my protagonists when paraphrasing their claims or explaining their views. This might make the study a little more difficult to read, at least until the reader has mastered the various different terms used, but it is necessary to proper hermeneutic sensitivity and hopefully allows my prose to convey something more of the feel and spirit of the world(s) it describes than might otherwise have been the case. I have also included some of the key linguistic transitions in my account, primarily because they are an important part of the story I am telling but also partly because I hope that this will increase the intelligibility of the story to those not yet 'in the know'.

# 1 Social movements, SMOs and fields of contention

I have stated that the primary focus of this study is the UK field of psychiatric contention between 1950 and 2000. In this brief chapter I will define in more detail what I mean by 'field of contention' and by the related concepts 'social movement' and 'social movement organisation' (SMO). My understanding of each of these concepts is derived from a critical dialogue with the ideas of Zald and McCarthy (1994). As representatives of the 'resource mobilisation' (RM) approach to social movement analysis, Zald and McCarthy are often criticised and dismissed in contemporary social movement analysis. Much of the criticism is justified in my view and I have added my own contribution to their critique (Crossley 2002a). Beyond the problems, however, there is something appealing about their model which makes it a good place to start thinking about 'social movements' and more particularly 'fields of contention'. We need to reconstruct their ideas but they provide an instructive point of departure. I begin, therefore, with Zald and McCarthy.

## Zald and McCarthy's field model

For Zald and McCarthy (1994) a 'social movement' is a vague current of collective sentiment within some part of society which expresses a demand for either change or resistance to change. There might be a feeling amongst some members of the general population, for example, that an activity of state, such as a war, is unacceptable. That would be a 'social movement' by this minimalist definition.

In addition, Zald and McCarthy continue, we sometimes find sentiments and demands which oppose those of a social movement. Other members of the population, for example, might think that war is justified and that opposition to the war is itself wrong for reasons, of being unpatriotic. This, in Zald and McCarthy's terminology, is a 'counter-movement'. Counter-movements oppose whatever it is that movements call for. They call for something different and usually something opposite. Thus we have both pro-choice and anti-abortion movements, fascists and anti-fascists, pro- and anti-hunting lobbies etc. I will be challenging the notion that contention between competing currents of opinion always breaks down into 'pro' and 'anti' camps later, and I will be suggesting that the concept of counter-movements is problematic for this reason. For present purposes, however, let's stick with these terms.

Zald and McCarthy do not clarify the nature of these sentiments and demands but I suggest, in opposition to what I think they would suggest, given their underlying theoretical orientation,[1] that we can think of them in terms of a communicative model. Social agents form opinions by means of interaction with others, both in their personal social networks, in institutional networks such as the church or workplace and by way of the broadcast networks[2] of the mass media. Interactions and the wider networks they comprise are the means by which ideas are both generated and passed on so as to become collective in the manner of a social movement.

Movements and counter-movements are of less interest to Zald and McCarthy, however, than the SMOs which take shape within them and which 'carry' them. Social movements, as Zald and McCarthy define them, do not and cannot do very much. They are not agents or actors (see Melucci 1989). In order for their sentiments to be expressed and translated into action they must be taken up by SMOs. Zald and McCarthy's model of SMOs is quite explicitly economic in inspiration. The relationship of SMOs to movements is one of 'supply' to 'demand'. Movements 'demand' expression and action, SMOs supply that expression and action in return for some form of 'payment', whether in the form of the symbolic support and recognition of '*adherents*', who share the view of an SMO, or the more material contributions of '*constituents*', who donate money and other tangible resources and who may become directly involved in the actions organised by SMOs. As in economic markets, this relationship can be either supply or demand led and will often involve an element of both. The formation of SMOs is often a response by political entrepreneurs to pre-existing problems (supply is generated to meet pre-existing demand). Equally, however, political entrepreneurs and their SMOs can seek to generate demand by trying to sell a problem and their solution to it. In either case, however, SMOs seek to draw individuals from the general population into their pool of adherents, and they seek to draw adherents into their pool of constituents.

Any social movement, Zald and McCarthy continue, will tend to generate more than one SMO. Thus, within environmentalism, to name only the most obvious, we have *Greenpeace, Friends of the Earth, Earth First!, Reclaim the Streets* and *The Earth Liberation Front*. Zald and McCarthy refer to these clusters as industries, arguing both that SMOs within industries compete with one another for resources and support and that this dynamic of interaction and competition is crucial to a proper understanding of contentious politics. 'All of the SMOs of a social movement industry', they argue, 'must be seen as part of *an interacting field*' (Zald and McCarthy 1994, 120, my emphasis). And it is this *field* which should form the central point in analysis.

Extending this point Zald and McCarthy argue, first, that there is competition among industries in what they call 'the movement sector'. The feminist industry, for example, must compete with the environmental and mental health industries for a finite pool of resources and support. Potential constituents have limited resources and cannot donate to every SMO or even to SMOs representing every worthy movement 'industry' or cause. They must be selective and this pressure upon them generates pressure between SMOs and industries who must compete to be selected. Second, they argue that the movement sector itself competes with the public, private and voluntary sectors of the economy. Agents who might give their resources to an SMO might also spend those resources on private goods, such as consumer durables, for example, or these resources might be absorbed through increased taxation within the public sector. How the sector and its component industries and SMOs fare is dependent upon its relationship to these other sectors. This links movement activism into the wider economic dynamics of society. Zald and McCarthy argue, for example, that there is evidence to suggest that movement activity increases during periods of affluence, and they seek to explain this by arguing that resources tend to be used for essential purchases in the private and public sectors during times of economic hardship, tending only to be freed up for the 'luxury' of donating to movements during periods of economic upturn. Figure 1.1 maps out the various successive layers of SMOs, industries and sectors described by Zald and McCarthy.

Underlying this model is the key claim of the RM approach to social movement analysis; namely, that political mobilisation presupposes a mobilisation or utilisation of scarce resources. That is why SMOs pursue constituents. Furthermore, this claim has the important implication that

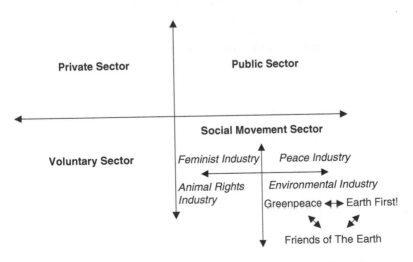

*Figure 1.1* Zald and McCarthy's model illustrated (and simplified).

political mobilisation (or at least successful mobilisation) is said to be dependent upon resource flows and thus to fluctuate with the fluctuations in resource flows. When the resource flow into an SMO, industry or the movement sector more generally increases, we can expect levels of contention to rise. When the flow dries up, so too will the contention.

Although I believe that RM theorists overestimate the significance of resource flows, they clearly have a point. We certainly need to consider resource mobilisation when we start to think about how we might explain the dynamics of contentious politics. What I find most interesting about the work of Zald and McCarthy, however, is their concept of fields. The concept of fields of interacting SMOs, linking to and competing for adherents and constituents is very persuasive in my view and forms the basis of my own concept of 'fields of contention'. It identifies an irreducible level of contentious politics, both in the concept of SMOs and the field constituted through their interaction. Insofar as SMOs have specific procedures for making and executing decisions we may, following Hindess (1988), grant them a status as ('minimal')[3] agents in their own right but this does not commit us to a view, much criticised in the literature, of 'movements' as collective actors or subjects (see Melucci 1989 for a critique of this view), not least because SMOs are not movements and, in any case, are situated in a field of social relations and interactions. It is this field which is our primary focus of analysis. The field, moreover, is irreducible and relational. The action of each agent within it, whether an individual, an SMO or some other organisational actor, responds to and anticipates the actions of at least some of the others, who do the same, such that no agent can be understood independently of the processual and interactive dynamics of the field as a whole. In addition, Zald and McCarthy encourage a dissection of contentious politics which the notion of 'movements' sometimes obscures. Whilst drawing 'the whole' into focus they simultaneously identify the division of labour and competitive tensions between its constituent parts. If the whole is greater than the sum of its parts this is only in virtue of the interdependencies and interactive dynamics between them. The moment one becomes acquainted with a movement, the existence of these 'parts' is often obvious but Zald and McCarthy are relatively rare in seeking to explore their interdependency.

There are problems with the model, however. I have spelled these out in detail elsewhere (Crossley 2002a). Here I will outline a few key problems. They come in three batches. The first relates to the economism of the model, the second to questions of culture and the third to issues of structure.

## The problem of economism and rational action

The market model evoked by Zald and McCarthy offers an image of individual entrepreneurs appealing to the demands or generating demand from a mass of individual consumers. This is problematic on a number of levels.

In the first instance it overlooks the importance, in at least some cases, of social networks. Here, the example of the black civil rights movement in the United States, is illustrative. The early SMOs of the movement grew out of community networks which were rooted in black churches and colleges and often preserved the organisational hierarchies (e.g. ministers as activist leaders) and cultural forms (e.g. hymn singing and hand holding) of those communities. Moreover, these SMOs sought 'block recruitment' from amongst congregational and student bodies, rather than individual recruits. Networks rather than individuals were the key 'building blocks' of this movement. This is not true of all movements, of course. One need only open a national newspaper for evidence of SMOs, such as *Greenpeace*, making appeals to individuals for money and support. And there is evidence that these professional 'mail order' SMOs have increased their 'market share' in recent years (Putnam 2000). Indeed Zald and McCarthy themselves make this case. However, we should at least be aware that the individualistic assumptions of Zald and McCarthy's model do not always hold, and we should be aware of a need to be able to think in more collective and relational ways.

Second, the idea of economic rationality, which, in the guise of rational action theory (RAT), guides Zald and McCarthy's model, is deeply problematic (Crossley 2002a, Feree 1992, Hindess 1998). It is difficult to deny that there is an element of truth to RAT. It is to the advantage of activists to pursue and use scarce resources in an efficient manner and most will tend to do so. Moreover, human action is purposive. It pursues goals. If one defines 'goals' as 'rewards' then much human action is, by definition, the pursuit of 'rewards'. The RAT model pushes this too far, however, claiming that 'rewards' are necessarily individual, selfish, material and stable over time – none of which is necessarily true (see Crossley 2002a). Moreover, it tends to ignore the role of interpretation in cognition and to presuppose, unrealistically, both 'perfect' information and extremely refined mechanisms of information processing, priority setting, strategising and tactical deliberation on behalf of social agents. This is problematic on many levels and fails to account for much of what we find in social movements. Indeed it fails to account for much of what Zald and McCarthy refer to in their own model. The selfish materialism of the approach, for example, fails to explain the often principled and altruistic demands of social movements: for example, humane treatment of animals, protection of the planet for the sake of future generations and the welfare of fellow human beings in distant societies. Why would selfish materialists be bothered about such ends? Furthermore, in their discussion of 'constituents' Zald and McCarthy accord a high priority to those who contribute resources to movements on the basis of conscience ('conscience constituents'). This is hardly rational economic behaviour!

We could push the point further by considering some of the considerable acts of self-sacrifice made by activists. From suicide bombers and hunger strikers through tunnelers and tree house dwellers[4] to the nameless many who stuff envelopes for 'lost causes', social movement activism throws up numerous examples of agents who give a great deal without much expectation of reward, certainly not in a material sense. Some RAT advocates deflect such criticism, claiming to find 'profit' in self-sacrifice, but their defences make the theory circular, as any goal becomes profitable and selfish, by definition. The further consequence of this is that the testable aspect of the theory, one of its virtues, celebrated by many of its advocates, is lost too (Crossley 2002a).

I suggest that we abandon RAT. We should stick with the idea that resources are important and will therefore often be sought after. We should also stick with the idea that human action pursues goals and, under most circumstances, seeks to maximise 'goods' and minimise 'bads'. But we should avoid carrying that to the absurd lengths of RAT. And we should allow ourselves a model of human agency which is richer and includes the many obvious human attributes and tendencies (socially generated and/or shaped in many cases) ignored by RAT including interpretation, conscience and even a sense of humour.

For similar reasons, I suggest that we relax the definition of SMOs suggested by Zald and McCarthy. Any large social movement involves multiple discrete networks, groups and organisations but by no means all of them conform to the model of economically rational organisation suggested by Zald and McCarthy (1994), and we overlook much of what is interesting about them if we assume that they do. I would rather think of an SMO as any group, network, organisation or collective project which has a discrete identity within a field of contention; that is, a collective formation that either thinks of itself as distinct or is recognised and known as such in the field. Usually this will be a named collective but often it will not be a 'rational' organisation, in the utilitarian sense. Indeed, in some cases it will involve collectives whose members strive to organise themselves in ways which depart from and resist the assumptions of a rational economic or political model.

## Cultures of contention

In some of their work Zald and McCarthy concede that they are too economistic. We need a more cultural model they suggest:

> Although we think the parallel with economic processes is striking, we should remember that there are differences. In particular, competition for dominance amongst SMOs is often for symbolic dominance, for defining the terms of social movement action. Social movement leaders are seeking symbolic hegemony. At some point social movement analysis must join with cultural and linguistic analysis if it is to understand fully co-operation and conflict in its socially specific forms.
>
> (Zald and McCarthy 1994, 180)

I couldn't agree more. Zald and McCarthy do not develop this aspect of their argument, however. We must. We need to be mindful that interaction within fields is generative of a movement discourse and culture; that is, of norms, identities, symbols, frames, typifications and a range of stories and sacred texts which identify heroes, villains, promised lands etc. This is not to say that members of a field agree about such matters but, as Bourdieu (1993) says in his conception of fields, they at least agree sufficiently to have something to disagree about. We need to be mindful of this cultural dimension in our investigation of fields of contention, following through on what Zald and McCarthy fail to deliver. I address this further in Chapter 2.

## Structure

A further problem with Zald and McCarthy's model is their failure to iden-tify that and how network patterns take shape within fields which structure those fields and which, potentially at least, have significant effects. I agree with Zald and McCarthy that SMOs interact and that these interactions are constitutive of (what I call) fields of contention but I want to take this fur-ther, following the lead of DiMaggio and Powell (1983), by noting that this does not entail every SMO interacting with every other SMO. Certain SMOs interact with certain others. More to the point, SMOs will interact in certain ways, giving rise to certain forms of relationship, with certain of their fellow SMOs, relating to others in other ways and perhaps not really relating at all to others still. Potentially there may be a great deal of fluidity involved here. I have used the term 'interaction' alongside 'relationship' in an attempt to indicate that relationships have to be 'done' and can be 'undone'. New rela-tionships form; old ones sometimes die out. They are always 'in process'. Indeed a field is itself a process. It is always in motion, with both SMOs and the patterns of relationships between them in a state of flux. However, rela-tively durable patterns of relationships can emerge in fields which are con-sequential in their own right and which give rise to broader network patterns or structures which are also significant. Our concept of fields of contention, I contend, needs to include these 'structures-in-process'.

Two types of structure are particularly important. First, there are struc-tures of positive links. By 'positive' I mean two things. In the first instance I mean relationships where something specifiable happens and where par-ties mutually affect one another: perhaps information is shared, resources are exchanged, pacts or temporary coalitions are formed etc. I would also include in this situations where SMOs enjoy overlapping membership, where members of different SMOs are friends or where representatives meet up at common events or committees under conditions where, perhaps inadvertently, they affect and/or pass things on to one another. Such rela-tionships may involve a great deal of negotiation and management, in Goffman's (1959) sense, and one can imagine that the significance which each party has for the other will be of great importance in relation to what happens in the relationship. However, this does not mean that parties to a relationship only affect others in intended ways or even ways they are aware of. The second meaning of positive refers more specifically to network structure. I mean that the pattern of positive links between SMOs and the wider network structure it gives rise to is of interest and relevance to us.

To illustrate this I have mapped two network structures. Figure 1.2 is a graph representing URL links between 22 contemporary mental health websites, most of which represent SMOs (the sample is not identical to the sample of SMOs discussed elsewhere in this study). Figure 1.3 is a graph representing the relationships, as known to me, between: first, my 35 interviewees (numbered 1–35, but not in accordance with the numbering used elsewhere in the book); second, a number of named 'stars' of psychiatric contention who are discussed in the book and third, a number of 'missing links' whom I would like to have interviewed but could not (labelled A–D). My intention in mapping these networks is purely illustrative. I want to demonstrate what I mean by network structure. There are many methodological issues and flaws which would have to be addressed if I intended to draw substantive conclusions about these structures for anything other than illustrative purposes. However, it is clear, I hope, that structures do emerge in both cases, which have specifiable properties and, one can hypothesise,

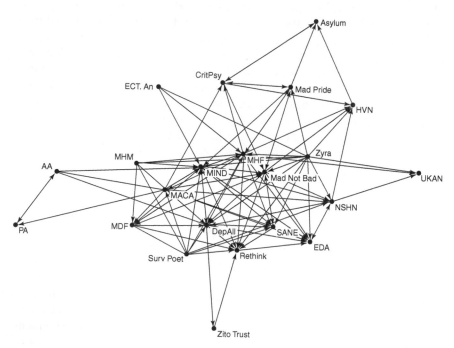

*Figure 1.2* URL links between mental health sites.

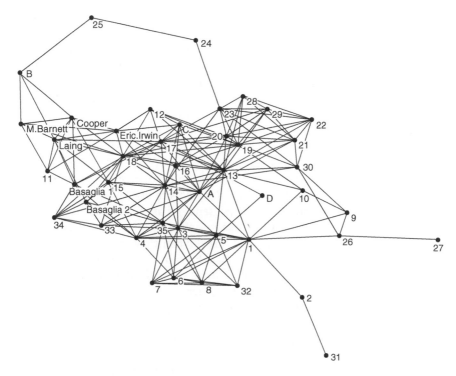

*Figure 1.3* A network of activist links.

concrete effects. To expand the illustration I will briefly discuss and dissect Figure 1.2 in greater detail.

A preliminary warning is necessary. URL links between websites have the great advantage, from the point of view of network analysis, of being both relatively unambiguous (one site either links directly to another or it doesn't) and being relatively easy to research. One can survey the links between a small sample of websites in an afternoon from the comfort of one's office. That is why I chose URL links for my illustration. However, like any other sort of relationship, URL links have a limited and bounded significance. Indeed, in the case of URL links one might argue that, for the most part, nothing much happens at this interface between sites/SMOs. For the sake of this analysis, therefore, I am going to take URL links to be proxies for a whole range of different types of relationship. There is absolutely no justification for doing this other than for illustration. If I seriously believed that URL links are good proxies for other types of relationships, you would have good reason to question my judgement. But I don't. I just want to illustrate a point and need an example.

The first obvious point to make with respect to the graph in Figure 1.2 is that it is possible to find a pathway of connecting links between any two points on it. Every point on the graph, by however circuitous a route, is linked to every other point. In the language of network analysis we say that the graph is 'connected' and consists of a single 'component' (Scott 1991). This observation is actually not as straightforward as it might first appear because the graph is a 'directed' graph (ibid.); that is, it does not record the presence or absence of a simple link between any two sites but rather records both whether a given site connects to another site and whether that other site connects back to the first. In the case of our example, this allows for the fact that some sites may be linked to by other sites which they do not themselves link to. The *Zito Trust*, located at the bottom/centre of the graph, for example, is listed as a link on the site of the *Depression Alliance* (DepAll) but does not reciprocate this link on its own site. Conversely, its site contains a link to *Rethink* but the *Rethink* site does not link back to it. This is indicated on the graph by the presence or absence of arrowheads on the connecting lines. Technically these connecting lines are referred to as 'edges' when they are undirected and 'arcs' when they are directed.

Network analysis does not have to work with 'directed graphs'. In fact, many of the more sophisticated procedures of analysis cannot accommodate direction. They assume that there either is a link between two sites or there isn't. Direction can be significant when we are considering the question of whether any one 'node' (the technical term for the points connected by the arcs/edges on a graph) can be reached from any other, however, as direction affects this. If the *Zito Trust* remained linked to *Rethink*, for example, but no site actually linked to it, then one would not be able to reach it from any of the other sites. Whether we could still refer to our graph as connected and as a single component in this case is too complicated an issue to deal with here but thankfully it doesn't arise as the *Depression Alliance*, as noted, links to the *Zito Trust* and we have an uncomplicated case of a connected graph.

The connection of the graph and its consisting in a single component is important because it indicates the potential, if these connections were communicative connections, for total diffusion. That is to say, any idea, innovation, norm or resource originating in one region of the graph might realistically pass through to all SMOs. This is no guarantee of homogeneity in the field because SMOs might reject the ideas and innovations passing through to them. However, it increases the chances that they will share a common focus to agree and disagree about. If the graph was divided into two or more components, there would be a greater possibility that groups in the different components were attending to quite different issues. Similarly, within a single component there is a greater likelihood that each node will at least know of every other node, because the name of each will tend to 'get around'.

It might be tempting to equate the issue of connectedness with cohesion. On one level, considering what I have said, this is probably so. If each party is aware of the others they can and will orient to the others and orient to the ways in which they anticipate the others will orient towards them. In addition, as noted, ideas pass around in a connected network, even if they are subject to disagreement from some quarters, and this lends the field a degree of cohesion. However, as the reference to disagreement indicates, this is not pre-emptive of conflict. Having greater of knowledge of others and their ideas does not necessarily lessen disagreement. Indeed, in many respects it is a pre-condition of it. The most we can say is that parties know better what they are disagreeing about and who they are disagreeing with.

The second network property we can consider is 'density'. Density is a measure of the number of connections in a network expressed as a fraction of the number of possible connections. In our network, for example, we have 22 nodes. Because the graph is directed, this means that there could be a total of 462 connections between them. There aren't, however, there are 117. The density of the network therefore is $117/462 = 0.25$. The maximum density score is 1, when the actual number of connections is equal to the total possible number: for example, $462/462 = 1$.

It is often difficult to attach meaning to density scores, not least because, for many reasons, they are not comparable across networks and we therefore cannot say whether a density score is low or high (ibid.). In our case, however, I would say that the density is low and that this is significant. URL links are 'cheap'. Very little effort is required to set them up and maintain them. Consequently every node could conceivably connect to every other. Indeed, many of the sites in the sample have more than 22 connections (because they connect to sites outside of the sample). A low density score therefore indicates either that, contrary to what was said above, the SMOs in the sample are largely unaware of one another's existence, which seems unlikely, or that they have been selective in their choice of who to link to and have, in many cases, chosen not to connect to one another.

A low density will tend to slow down diffusion processes. Whatever moves through a network tends to have to do so by more circuitous routes. This might also increase the possibility that information is lost along the way. In addition, it might also lessen cohesion. If we assume, for example, that every relationship in a network involves a degree of interdependency and thus what Elias (1979) calls a 'power balance', that is, we assume that each node exerts a controlling influence on every other, then we would expect a high level of cohesion in high density networks as each node is subject to the same controlling influences. As density decreases, however, although this depends upon the pattern we are left with, there is a greater chance that different parts of the graph will be subject to different controlling influences, such that overall cohesion is reduced. There are a number of outlying nodes and regions on our graph, for example, which would assumedly be subject to less or at least different controlling influences than more central nodes, if the arcs in our graph represented relations of (reciprocal) control.

Another noteworthy property of the graph is 'centrality'. Centrality is a key concept in social network analysis and is defined and measured in a number of different ways. Some definitions focus upon the centrality of specific nodes within the graph, whilst other focus upon the overall level of centralisation of the graph itself. And within this broad distinction there are further distinctions. The centrality of specific nodes, for example, is sometimes measured in terms of their number of connections ('degrees'), the best-connected nodes being deemed the most central. This is sometimes called 'degree centrality'. In other instances, by contrast, the centrality of nodes is measured by reference to the extent to which a node lies between and connects other nodes and regions of the graph. One can imagine a situation, for example, in which a single node connects what are effectively two sides of a graph; the node may have relatively few connections but those connections play a key role in holding the two sides of the graph together and this makes the node central.

In order to illuminate the significance of centrality let us consider degree centrality in our graph. For the sake of convenience, bearing in mind that our graph is directed, I will measure this in terms of the number of positive connections that each site receives from other sites (its 'indegree'). The values are presented in the graph in Figure 1.4. The values vary between 1 and 14, which is a broad range. Some sites are clearly much more central than others. We might say that they enjoy a higher level of social capital relative to the

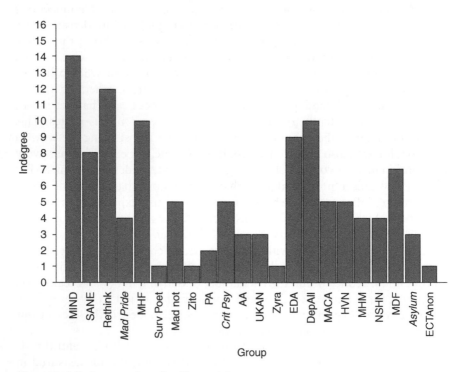

*Figure 1.4* Indegree values for Figure 1.2.

field, which they can perhaps draw upon in their campaigning activities, if necessary. MIND has 14 'friends' to call upon, for example, where *Survivor Poetry* (Surv Poet) has only 1.

In addition these more central sites, or rather the SMOs they represent, are more likely to be better informed of what is going on in the field, because they have a larger and more diverse range of potential sources of information. For both of these reasons we might hypothesise that their efficacy is enhanced by their position in the field. At the same time, however, high degree centrality might generate constraints for those SMOs who enjoy it. Norms of obligation between connected parties can act as a constraint, for example, and a higher number of connections increases the number of obligations. Moreover, it increases the likelihood that obligations will be competing, if not conflicting, thus constricting an SMO's possibilities for acting. Furthermore, well-connected and well-known players are less able to play their cards close to their chests or to secure the strategic advantages attaching to secrecy and surprise. They are more closely scrutinised by others and their lines of connection are potentially channels for significant leaks of information. Both of these factors might decrease the efficacy of central nodes. However, the point I am trying to make is not really about increased or decreased efficacy. It is a matter of indicating how position within the network structure of a field of contention is potentially significant. Different positions in the pattern of relations generate different opportunities and constraints.

Finally, note that we can identify distinct regions in a network, set out from the rest of the network. In our graph, for example, at the top we find a triangle, set apart from the main 'pack', involving the *Asylum* journal, the *Hearing Voices Network* (HVN), the *Mad Pride* group and the *Critical Psychiatry Network*. As the names suggest, these are some of the more radical sites/SMOs in the field. There are other radical sites, of course, most of which connect directly to this triangle but some of which also connect to less radical and more conservative sites. Nevertheless, our analysis might be drawn to this specific region and we might expect projects emerging in this region of the network to be different from those elsewhere. The field is differentiated and a network analysis allows us to identify and map that differentiation.

Much the same type of analysis might be made with respect to the individual activists identified in Figure 1.3. I will not repeat the illustrative analysis. Note, however, that many of the links between individuals in that graph cut across SMOs such as those identified in Figure 1.2, partly because some individuals are members of more than one SMO, partly because friendships develop across organisational barriers. Links between activists can, in this respect, be regarded as links between SMOs. The latter are linked by virtue of the links of their individual members. At the same time, however, multiple memberships indicate how the boundaries of SMOs are often quite blurred and cross-organisational friendships indicate that informal boundaries within a field might be drawn in different ways to formal boundaries. Indeed, at certain points in my research I sometimes wondered whether many SMOs weren't really just convenient labels that different clusters of activists within a broader network occasionally drew upon to give focus and identity to a project, the underlying network being the more interesting and important phenomena. SMOs come and go, to some extent, whilst the underlying network that generates them and provides their membership is more stable (though, of course, also always 'in process'). I will revisit this point.

We could push our network analysis further, deepening it and introducing more network properties and measures. I have said enough, however, to establish that fields are structured in accordance with the pattern of connections between SMOs within them and that this structure is potentially consequential. I will not be using formal network analysis very much in the study, partly because of the unavailability of the necessary data. What I am more concerned about, however, is the way of thinking, relationally and structurally, that its concepts encourage. Patterns of relations are important. We must set this within time. We need to think of structure-in-process, of connections being made anew, remade and broken through on-going processes of interaction. But the structure is as important as the process.

The second type of structure that I discuss relates to what network theorists call 'structural equivalence' (Scott 1991). This entails that nodes in a network enjoy relationships with a similar set of further nodes, even if they have no significant relationship to one another. This might entail two or more SMOs having connections to the same set of other SMOs, even though they have no relation to one another. Alternatively, it may involve SMOs having relationships to the same funding bodies, pools of adherents, constituents, elites, allies etc. even if they enjoy no significant relations with one another. A hypothetical case of this is represented in Figure 1.5. Equivalence is significant because it configures SMOs in a potentially competitive situation, at least if there is a limited supply of the resources they want from their common connections.

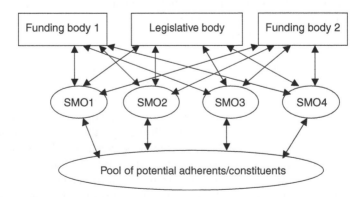

*Figure 1.5* Structural equivalence between SMOs.

One SMO's gain may be another's loss. DeMaggio and Powell argue that this can generate a tendency for organisations to become increasingly similar, especially when there is uncertainty in an action situation. Each SMO mirrors the others in an effort to avoid losing out on the potential profit of a particular strategy. I have found evidence of this in my study but, as I argue in subsequent chapters, I have also found that structurally equivalent groups sometimes seek to distinguish themselves from one another and carve out a niche, as Durkheim's (1964) and Simmel's (1950) respective arguments on the division of labour would predict. Moreover, in some cases I have encountered SMOs who are mindful of the 'silly' competitive situation they are in who have attempted (in different ways and with varying degrees of success) to collaborate to avoid this problem. In all cases, however, structural equivalence generates a significant 'field effect' of which we should be mindful. Again the agent or SMO cannot be properly understood independently of the field in which they are involved and we must attend to network structures.

## Defining fields of contention

Adopting this important idea of structural equivalence necessitates that we define fields of contention as involving not just SMOs and their adherents and constituents but also all relevant actors, organisations and institutions to whom SMOs might be connected: for example potential funding bodies, government departments, journalists and other media agents, solicitors, even the police and security services, who can be very significant players in the protest game. This effectively prevents us from drawing a sharp dividing line between any field of contention and the wider society to which it belongs but that is important because struggles are never cut off from wider society and tracing links in this way allows us to study the interaction of SMOs with the wider world, without posing, as I have elsewhere, a problematic distinction between 'internal' and 'external' accounts. The network of agents involved in a field of contention is a sub-network of the wider network of a national and even international society and is best considered as such if we want to understand contentious politics in its proper social context. Having said that, we need to draw boundaries around fields of contention if our project is to be manageable and meaningful, and we should do this, in my view, by seeking to identify and include all key players in relation to a specific area of contention (in this case psychiatry and mental health), whether they be SMOs, professional bodies, funding bodies or any of a range of other relevant agencies.

## Social movements?

Where does this talk of fields leave the notion of 'social movements'? Zald and McCarthy, having used the notion of social movements to set up their argument, seem to drop it. Sentiment pools are still referred to in their work, in the form of pools of adherents and constituents, but the term 'social movement' is seldom used by them and its place within their final schema is unclear. I want to keep the concept, however, because I believe that it still serves a useful discriminatory function. Within any given field of contention, both over time and at any particular point in time, one can find different discourses and demands, each of which might be represented by a number of distinct SMOs. 'Social movements' captures these different currents. This might be a matter of what Zald and McCarthy (1994) call 'movements' and 'counter-movements' but, as indicated earlier, distinctions do not necessarily break down in this binary fashion. There may be more than two currents of discourse–demand in a field at any point of time and these currents will not necessarily stand in direct opposition to one another. I noted in the Introduction, for example, that at certain points in the history of the field of psychiatric contention we find SMOs representing anti-psychiatry, civil rights, the 'patients' movement' and what I called 'anti-anti-psychiatry'. In most cases, moreover, there was more than one SMO representing each of these movements. Although I am sceptical with respect to the notion of counter-movements, I would like to preserve the notion of 'social movements' as a term for SMOs, adherents and constituents who cluster around particular discursive-demand currents within a field. Distinguishing discourses–demands and their 'movements' is inevitably an imprecise business. The dividing line between discourses is often blurred and each individual agent involved in a field assimilates a discourse differently, such that individual expressions of the same discourse tend to vary. It can be a useful, heuristically, to make distinctions, however, particularly when we are looking at different and competing historical waves of mobilisation within a field. I offer 'social movements' and their 'discourses' in this heuristic spirit.

## Conclusion

In this chapter I have defined three key concepts. By 'social movements', I refer to relatively diffuse currents of demand and discourse. Movements are 'carried' by SMOs but they also involve pools of adherents and constituents who 'donate' both symbolic and material resources (including sometimes time and effort) to SMOs. Any movement may be carried by more than one SMO. SMOs are defined by Zald and McCarthy as economically rational organisations who seek resources from their constituents. I take a much broader definition. SMOs are any collectivity or project within a field which has a relatively distinct identity therein and elects to act on behalf of the demands of a particular movement, embodying its discourse. They are not necessarily economically rational, nor are they necessarily preoccupied with amassing material resources (although many are, to some degree, and all need material resources to engage in sustained actions). And they are not necessarily preoccupied with amassing adherents and constituents (although again some level of support is often necessary to success). Small direct actions cells are SMOs, as are large donation-seeking organisations, and the 'experiments in living' discussed by Alberto Melucci (1989).

Fields of contention are the social spaces generated by interaction between SMOs, within and across social movements, who converge around common areas of concern (whether in agreement or disagreement), and also between these SMOs and other agents whose actions have a significant impact upon these SMOs: groups of (potential) constituents and adherents, professional bodies, funding bodies, government, journalists etc. These fields are always 'in process', like society itself. They are constantly in motion by virtue of the interactions which constitute them. However, this does not preclude the possibility of structure or, as I have called it, 'structure-in-process'. We can identify patterns within the flux of interaction, some of which will be relatively durable and some of which, whether or not they are durable, will have effects. In part, to pick up a point I have only hinted at here, this structure arises out of the differential levels of resources available to distinct SMOs. Some are better resourced than others, although this is always relative to particular, different types of resources. In addition, however, it is also a matter of emergent network structures, which change over time but which nevertheless have an impact for the extent of their duration.

Finally I have indicated that interaction within fields is culturally generative. Norms, narratives, discourses, identities etc. emerge, mutate and diffuse in this context. In part these cultural elements express and effect conflicts. They do not effect a 'common culture and value system', in the functionalist sense. At the same time, however, they do generate and emerge from common reference points, affording agreement over what is to be disagreed about and what the rules of engagement are. And they can lend the field a sense of being a social world in its own right. When I first began to research the field of psychiatric contention, for example, I was aware of a vocabulary and common sense of history amongst many activists, even those in conflicting movements and SMOs, which it was necessary for me to grasp before I could properly begin my research. We might call this the culture of the field of contention or the culture of contention.

# 2 A value-added model of mobilisation

Having outlined my model of fields, SMOs and movements in the previous chapter, I turn in this chapter to a model of the factors which help to explain their emergence, form, survival and decline. Before I introduce this model, however, a brief qualification is necessary. Protest, resistance, political contention and social movements are often cited in sociological studies as indications of agency; of the fact that members of society are not completely duped by dominant ideologies nor overwhelmed by power; that they do not simply go with the flow but are capable of assessing their situations and acting in ways which pursue change. Complementing this, there has been an interesting turn in recent US movement analysis away from the causal models of mobilisation which predominated for a long time, towards an approach which focuses upon mechanisms, processes, interdependencies, interactions and relations (see especially McAdam *et al.* 2001, for a more general discussion, see Abbott 2001). Movements unfold as dynamic processes in this view, as agents make sense of self, others and world in complex interaction processes which defy linear and causal models. My field model, as outlined in Chapter 1, is very much informed by this recent turn.

If we take these matters of agency, process and interaction seriously, as I do, then sociological models, such as the one discussed in this chapter, can seem clumsy and inappropriate. They separate out elements of a story which, in the context of the story, are mingled, simultaneously interfering with and misrepresenting its apparent temporal structure. They reduce processes to 'boxes' or variables, deleting human work and interaction. They simplify and they may even appear to squeeze agency out of the picture. The best, most sensitive models cannot always avoid these problems.

Models play an important part in sociological analysis, however. I accept that they simplify. That is their job. The point of sociological analysis, like other forms of scientific analysis, is to clarify complex processes, simplifying them such that they are amenable to human understanding. Models are one of the ways in which this is achieved. They reduce complexity in order to increase comprehension. If they are understood in this spirit, as aids to understanding, and if we remain mindful of their complexity-reducing function, then there is no need to see models as problems. Moreover, there is no reason why we cannot use models *alongside more nuanced historical narratives which emphasise agency, interaction and process.*

On a more positive note, models afford the possibility of a degree of standardisation in analysis and thus comparison across cases. This is important on two counts. First, it allows us to build a general knowledge of social movements, beyond specific cases. Second, it enhances our analysis of any particular case by suggesting leads that we may follow, contrasts and similarities that we can contemplate and so on. Moreover, the level of generality encouraged by the model allows us to identify broad patterns and regularities that can get lost in the detail and particularity of focused narratives. They allow us to step back and view our case in a different light. Without this it is often very difficult to see the wood for the trees.

In short we need both narrative accounts, which are sensitive to agency, interaction and process, and theoretical models which abstract from the narrative flow seeking out key factors which shape its trajectory and render it comparable with other, similar narratives. In this book I attempt this combination but in the present chapter I am focusing specifically upon the theoretical model.

My model is a reconstructed version of Neil Smelser's (1962) value-added model of collective behaviour (see also Crossley 2002a). There are many problems with Smelser's model. Certainly I do not want to buy into his psychodynamic model of agency or his functionalist account of structure. And I want to strip out all traces of these elements as they manifest within his model. But there is a crucial insight in Smelser's model that no other theorist has articulated, which makes it invaluable. Moreover, this is an insight which allows it to incorporate many later insights of social movement theory, including the insights of writers who have been very critical of Smelser. Smelser's model is a useful 'junction box' for incorporating and connecting a variety of important insights from social-movement studies, old and new.

Smelser's conceptual map is different to my own. He posits a theory of 'collective behaviour', which includes a focus on what he calls norm and value-oriented social movements,[1] alongside crazes, panics and 'hostile outbursts', but he has no concept of SMOs or fields, at least not explicitly. His model can, however, incorporate this different conceptual mapping relatively easily, as I will show. And the payoff is, in my view, worth the effort required to bring it about.

## The value-added model

It seems obvious, *prima facie*, that movements and their SMOs generally oppose some state of affairs in the social world. The social world is not equally pleasing or rewarding for all people. It gives rise to a range of 'strains' or 'grievances' for some. And social movements and SMOs mobilise around these strains and grievances. SMOs express grievances, critique the conditions that give rise to strain and call for change. Or if change is the perceived cause of the problem, they call for a halt to change, for conservation or restoration of the *status quo ante*. One might be tempted, therefore, to seek to explain movements and SMOs by reference to grievances and strains. Strains and grievances are good *reasons* for mobilising, so perhaps they are also the causes, necessary and sufficient, of it? Much work in social movement studies has challenged this idea, suggesting that strains are not sufficient causes. Some even suggest that they may not be necessary.[2] There have been studies, for example, which have shown that variations in mobilisation rates over time do not correlate with variations in levels of objective hardship (e.g. Snyder and Tilly 1972). Such studies are far from conclusive because most definitions of strain in the literature suggest that it arises out of a mismatch between (inter)subjective expectations and objective conditions, rather than from objective hardships *per se*. It is not objective hardship which generates strain and subsequent mobilisation, the argument goes, but rather a breach of expectations that certain forms of hardship give rise to. There is therefore no reason to believe that levels of mobilisation will tally with levels of objective hardship because the latter may not tally with levels of strain. At a more general level, however, it is observed: (1) that political mobilisation often follows reform and improvement in living conditions (e.g. a period of increased affluence or a lifting of restrictions and repression); (2) that levels of hardship and grievance can remain constant in a situation whilst levels of mobilisation fluctuate; and (3) that levels of felt and expressed grievance can be relatively high without it necessarily leading to significant mobilisation (Crossley 2002a, Jenkins and Perrow 1977, McAdam 1982). Clearly there are further conditions, additional to strain, which are necessary if mobilisation is to occur. Much of the history of social-movement theory, at least in the United States between the 1970s and the 1990s, is a history of successive attempts to pinpoint those conditions (Crossley 2002a).

I have examined this history elsewhere and have argued that Smesler's value-added model of mobilisation provides the best framework for synthesising its insights (Crossley 2002a). Smelser's work is flawed in major respects and is almost universally rejected by movement scholars. He posits a very problematic conception of 'the growth and spread of generalised belief' (see later), which forms part of an equally problematic conception of human agency (Crossley 2002a). And his concept of 'structure' is also flawed (ibid.). His account is important, however, because he resisted the tendency, evident in much work both before and after, to identify a single cause for movement formation, suggesting a multifactoral, interactive and processual model instead.

Smelser borrows the idea of a value-added model from economics. Value-added models in economics stipulate how the different stages in a production process each contribute something unique and different to that process; raw materials are extracted, for example, then perhaps melted down and cast into 'parts', which are next painted, then assembled and so on. Value is added to the final product at each stage. Smelser argues that we need to think about collective behaviour in much the same way. Movements are not the product of a single cause but rather of interacting processes which contribute differently to their formation. Failure of any one process to meet the pre-requisites of mobilisation will result in a failure of mobilisation, or rather variation in the various processes will result in variation in the type of collective behaviour which emerges. Norm and value oriented social movements are two possible 'outcomes' of the interacting processes Smelser considers but other potential outcomes include: (1) riots and such 'hostile outbursts' as lynchings, (2) panic of various kinds, including 'moral panic' and (3) crazes. And of course these different types of collective behaviour can coexist and interact in a variety of ways. Concern over the environment, for example, might, in the right conditions, give rise simultaneously to social movements, panics, crazes and hostile outbursts of various kinds.

Where the value-added conditions which generate collective behaviour differ from those of economic production is, first, that they can fall into place in any order. Raw materials have to be extracted before they can be moulded, painted etc., but the value-added elements of social movement formation do not have a fixed temporal order. Sometimes X comes before Y and Y is the final trigger of mobilisation. Other times Y comes before X and X is the trigger. Much time has been wasted in social-movement studies by scholars trying to prove the causal primacy of their own pet X or Y, and the period between the early 1970s and the late 1990s was punctuated by a succession of fashions for largely monocausal explanations. Smelser offers a welcome relief from this and a wholly more convincing view. Second, the elements of his process, outlined below, are 'analytical'; that is to say, theoretically speaking there are always six distinct elements involved in mobilisation but practically speaking the same event, process or state of affairs may count more than once if it has different effects which correspond to the different analytic elements. A particular social change may generate strain, for example, whilst simultaneously enhancing 'conduciveness' (see later) and weakening the power of agents of control to stem an uprising (below). Smelser's six value-added elements are

1    structural conduciveness;
2    structural strain;
3    growth and spread of generalised belief;
4    precipitating factors;
5    mobilisation of participants for action and
6    operation of social control.

I will briefly discuss each of these in turn.

## Structural conduciveness

Any social action, whether it be individual or collective, oppositional or compliant, is shaped by structural features of the context in which it occurs. Dissidents in totalitarian and repressive states, for example, have little opportunity for overt protest and campaigning. Unless they feel they have sufficient support to mount a successful revolutionary struggle or are prepared to face imprisonment or death, they must conduct their struggles underground and must operate in ways which avoid bringing those struggles to the attention of the authorities. In some cases disaffected individuals may feel that the risks are too great to do anything at all. In a different vein, passengers on a sinking ship do not have the time to form an SMO to lobby the shipping company for better safety procedures. They are constrained to do what they can to survive the sinking – after which, when the structural conditions of their action have changed, they might think about campaigning. Particular forms of collective behaviour will only take shape, therefore, in conditions which are conducive to them. And new forms of collective behaviour, such as movement and SMO formation, may be triggered by a shift in conditions of structural conduciveness. If conditions become more conducive then movement mobilisation becomes more likely.

I noted above that many of Smelser's ideas have been rediscovered by subsequent social-movement theories. Structural conduciveness is a good example of this. Two of the key 'causes' of mobilisation cited in later movement theorising can be construed as examples of structural conduciveness. The most obvious is the idea of the 'political opportunity structure' (Crossley 2002a, Tarrow 1998). Protest and movement formation occur, according to proponents of this idea, when there is a perceived opening of opportunities in the political system: for example, when cracks appear in a regime or repression is lifted. The proliferation of oppositional SMOs in the former Soviet Union, following *Glasnost* and subsequent reforms, is often held up as a key example of this (Tarrow 1998). Moreover, opportunities are said to shape the form of political action. Comparative studies suggest, for example, that protests addressing the same issues take different forms in different societies. And this is interpreted in terms of the different structures of political opportunity in those societies (Kitschelt 1986). Different things are possible in different political contexts at different points in time.

The concept of political opportunity is important. However, along with other writers in the field, I believe that the concept of opportunity structures needs to be extended beyond the bounds of the polity (e.g. McAdam 1994). Social movement struggles in complex, differentiated societies can take place simultaneously in the courts, the media, parliament, the academic world, in economic markets etc. Each of these social fields offers variable and independent opportunities and constraints which shape collective behaviour in a variety of ways. We need to extend the notion of 'opportunity structures' to each of these domains and to all domains that might become implicated in contentious politics.

Opportunities are dependent, however, upon the resources of agents. To play the media, legal or academic game, for example, requires that one have the competence, status and contacts, not to mention finances, necessary to play that game effectively. Without these resources, opportunities are less likely and may not present themselves as meaningful possibilities. This resources factor, which I believe also falls under the rubric of 'structural conduciveness', was explored and championed in social movement studies by the Resource Mobilisation (RM) school to which Zald and McCarthy (1994), discussed in Chapter 1, belong (Crossley 2002a, Jenkins 1983). There is some controversy in the literature surrounding this school, much of which hangs on the fact that some RM theorists appear to suggest that protest by poor and powerless groups only happens when their cause is adopted by richer and more influential groups ('elite patronisation'), a claim which has been strongly challenged (McAdam 1982, Piven and Cloward 1979, 1992). However, this is only one claim of RM theory, not subscribed to by all, and there is an important kernel of truth in the more general claim of RM theorists that protest uses resources, is therefore resource dependent, and thus fluctuates in accordance with the fluctuations of resource flows. Some acts of protest, admittedly, require very little by way of resources. However, many do require resources and this is particularly true if isolated acts of resistance are to be transformed into sustained efforts to bring about change. It is for this reason that governments and agencies of social control strive to cut off the resource flows of terrorist groups. Without resources there is very little that these groups can do. The conduciveness of a particular structural context of action, therefore, is a function of the availability of relevant resources within it, in addition to the other opportunities and constraints it presents.

It is important to add that mobilisation itself alters conditions and perceptions of structural conduciveness. If an elite is under attack, for example, that makes it (or makes it appear) more vulnerable, thus encouraging further attacks. Political opportunity increases. In addition, different SMOs generate protest-relevant resources for one another. Alternative media groups, for example, generate channels of communication and publicity for other groups. Moreover, if there is a chance that one SMO will succeed in securing goods for one social group this may encourage the formation of further SMOs representing other groups who are frightened of 'falling behind'. Arguments of this kind have been used to explain what are variously referred to as 'cycles' or 'waves' of contention (McAdam 1995, Tarrow 1995, 1998, Traugott 1995). The concept of waves is based upon the observation that society periodically enters phases, such as the 'the Sixties', where both the number of SMOs and movements within it and the activity level of those SMOs and movements increases. The level of contention in society goes up. The term 'wave' or 'cycle' is employed in order to emphasise the statistically verified observation that the build up and wind down of such periods is graduated (see Traugott 1995). When plotted on a graph it is curved and thus wave-like. In other words, societies do not move from perfect calm to political crisis and back again in an instant (Tarrow 1995). The concept of waves is underdeveloped and arguably hampered by the rational action models that have been employed to flesh it out. However, the phenomenon captured by the concept is clearly significant in relation to a consideration of structural conduciveness and it is very relevant for this study, as my temporal focus includes 'the Sixties'.

## Structural strain

Strain is a complex phenomenon which could be explored at great depth. For the present purposes, however, let us say that in many cases it arises out of a mismatch between objective states of affairs and individual or shared expectations which bear upon them. It is the sense of frustration that agents experience when they lose control of their circumstances, when their hopes and beliefs are disappointed and/or they feel wronged. Groups who live in the lap of luxury may experience strain, from this point of view, if they expect more than they get. Conversely, as E.P. Thompson (1993) notes with respect to protest in eighteenth century England, dreadful conditions can fail to prompt strain if these conditions conform to the (low) expectations of those who must endure them.

Mismatch between expectations and reality, as Herbert Blumer (1969) argues, can be the effect of changes in expectations, reality or both, such that the same conditions might provoke strain in one era but not another, if expectations change. Moreover, Blumer notes that changes in expectations may be the effect of the activities of political 'agitators' (SMOs and their representatives) who encourage a rise in expectations in the hope that their lack of fulfillment will trigger strain and resentment.

In terms of the model discussed in Chapter 2, strain is an integral element of the demand that is constitutive of social movements. Demands emerge because social changes generate a misalignment of expectations and actualities which, in turn, generates strain, and because agents feel this strain and are keen to be relieved of it. Strain generates an emotional need and energy for action.

## The formation and spread of generalised beliefs

Exactly how the agent addresses a strain will depend upon a variety of factors, as the value-added model suggests, but one very crucial factor is their interpretation of it. If, for example, they attribute the cause of the strain to their own failings then their response might be to become depressed or to engage in some sort of self-harming behaviour. Alternatively, they might attribute the cause of their stress to an out-group of some sort, leading them to attack that out-group. Or they might attribute it to particular institutions in their society, in which case they might be led to join, form or support an SMO, perhaps taking part in organised protest. They become part of a social movement.

This is a crucial point but Smelser develops it via a crude psychoanalytic model which reduces processes of belief formation to such psychic mechanisms as 'wish fulfilment', 'projection' etc. Smelser (1962, 73) claims that this does not detract from the rationality of protest and social movements but it is difficult to accept this claim, particularly when elsewhere in his account he claims that collective behaviour 'short circuits' the social system and has a 'primitive', 'clumsy' and 'impatient' character. There is no room here for the possibility that agents may sometimes have a clearheaded analysis of their situation. More importantly, there is no sense of the (potential) rationality of the process whereby they arrive at their analysis: for example, of their deliberations, research and attempts to look at their situation from different points of view. Finally, there is little recognition of the inter-subjective nature of belief formation; that is, of the role of discussion and argument. Agents are not atoms and they do not arrive at their views and interpretations in a vacuum. They talk to one another and their views are formed and transformed by way of such interaction.

The initial response to this formulation, on behalf of many of Smelser's early critics, was to swing in the opposite direction, opting for a rational action model. However, this is equally if not more problematic (Crossley 2002a), and a newer generation of theorists have begun to explore different ways of thinking about cognition, interpretation and emotion. Goffman's (1974) ideas about 'framing' have been particularly singled out in this context. How agents respond to a situation, the argument goes, depends upon the way in which they frame that situation. Different framings bestow different meanings and thus invite or call for different responses. Moreover, as such, the framing process is crucial for SMOs wishing to secure adherents and constituents. Indeed much of the early social movements literature on framing was focused upon SMOs' attempts to draw in support and resources through framing strategies (Snow and Benford 1992, Snow *et al.* 1986). SMOs attempt to win support, it was argued, by way of framing activities which link their concerns and outlook to those of potential constituents (ibid.).

The concept of frames can be problematic, particularly if they are treated as static, unchanging, 'ready-made' aspects of culture, and if, as has happened, the concept is combined with models of the actor (such as the rational action model) which do not sit happily with it. Marc Steinberg (1995, 1999) has been particularly critical of the literature on framing for these reasons and has called for an alternative approach to issues of meaning and interpretation in political contention, based around what he calls 'discursive repertoires'. Discursive repertoires, he argues, build up in a context of struggle through dialogues both within and between the various parties involved. Moreover, they are not simply 'advertising strategies' for political positions, as some framing theorists have assumed of frames. They define reality for agents, particularly the key activists who use them to generate and maintain support – although, as Steinberg notes, they are also shaped by those central players' attempts to key into the perspectives of less or uninvolved players, so as to draw them into struggle. Steinberg's empirical account is impressive. However, used properly, as Goffman (1974) uses it, the concept of framing captures everything that he seeks to capture and perhaps more. Whilst frames can be mobilised and used cynically, like advertising materials, by agents who enjoy a reflective distance from them, they can equally emerge 'in the heat' of interaction, defining reality for those whose interactions, in turn, generate them. And they can slip in and out of place. Sometimes agents view the world through the lens of the frame. Other times they stand at a distance from frames, achieving a perspective on the frame that may be reflexive and self-critical or strategic and cynical. Moreover frames are always 'in process', changing as agents use them, innovate and improvise with them, pass them on to others etc. Finally, frames, from Goffman's point of view, are the product of human interaction. They emerge, take shape, diffuse and change within communicative exchanges between agents, as those agents absorb, respond to and anticipate the ideas and responses of those with whom they interact. In the context of contentious politics this might include interactions between: activists; activists and their opponents; activists and potential adherents/ constituents. Moreover, it will involve such communicative triangles as that which forms when both activists and their opponents seek to appeal to the same potential constituents. Such interactions may occasion cynicism and spin. However, as Blumer (1986) notes, attempts to persuade the unpersuaded and to out-argue opponents can induce a discipline, rigour and multi-perspectival aspect into argument which is of the essence of rationality, at least in its communicative sense (on communicative rationality see also Habermas 1991).

However, the concept 'frame' is too limited in my view. It is focused upon the work involved in constructing (framing) particular views of particular situations and is less applicable to, for example, the theories and ideologies that movement participants subscribe to or the narratives of a movement's history that circulate within it, orienting actions and identities. To accommodate these wider aspects, I will refer to movement discourses, which I define as broad complexes of ideas, vocabularies, frames, narratives, theories and ideologies that are operative within a specific movement community and that, to a large degree, define that movement community.

In terms of the model discussed Chapter 1, we are referring here to the discourses that are constitutive of specific social movements and which transform the vague dissatisfactions associated with social strain into concrete demands, which are also constitutive of social movements. Such discourses may emerge organically, in the hurly burly of everyday interaction, but journalists may also play a key role in shaping them as may also SMOs. SMOs respond to discourses and demands which pre-exist them but they are also sites where these discourses are worked over and modified, both through passionate debates and in the context of the development of more cynical 'framing' strategies. Moreover having 'fine tuned' discourses and demands, SMOs then pump them back into the general population in an effort to generate support and enlarge the movement to which they belong.

It might be instructive in this context to say a few words about 'cultures of contention'. Herbert Blumer (1969) is an important source in this context. He identifies a number of cultural/identity elements which may take shape in contexts of strain, arguing that movement formation and protest are much more likely if these elements emerge. Amongst the components that he lists are ideologies and tactics, both of which are important. For the moment, however, I want to single out the two other key components that Blumer mentions: '*esprit de corps*' and 'morale'. An *esprit de corps* is a feeling of group belonging and solidarity which operates at a pre-reflective and pre-linguistic level. The agent feels their self to be part of the group and experiences the group as a force which is greater and sometimes more important than their self. They experience a 'calling' from the group and a strong sense of obligation and duty in relationship to it. This *esprit de corps*, whilst by no means a necessary outcome of interaction, can sometimes be built up, according to Blumer, if interaction is intense and affectively charged. The intensity (fear, joy and power) of political demonstrations can engender it, as can collective singing and a range of group activities. Although he doesn't make the connection, McAdams' (1988) discussion of the biographical impact of 'freedom summer'[3] on those who took part describes this very well. He describes a 'freedom high' and collective fear which generated strong feelings of inter-dependence and a powerful bond between participants, which, in turn, had a lasting impact upon their life course and identity. Participation in 'high risk' activism gave rise to an *esprit de corps* which lasted for years and which many participants spent much time in their later lives seeking to recapture (ibid.).

Symbols, such as the CND sign, the swastika, the circled 'A' of the anarchists and the red flag, which are common in social movement politics, can also be important to this process, in Blumer's view, since they come to represent this shared feeling and become a condensed expression of it. The power of political, religious and nationalist symbols to trigger strong emotional responses (whether positive or negative) is clear evidence of this. The production of symbols is an important element in the process whereby agents build their sense of collective identity and belonging, their *esprit de corps*.

On top of this, at a more discursive level, Blumer discusses the role of 'saints', 'sinners', 'heroes', 'martyrs', 'myths' and 'sacred texts' in generating what he calls 'morale'. Groups pull together and make themselves into groups, he argues, by telling and sharing collective stories; stories which function to define a collective identity and shared situation for them. Ideology and tactics are necessary to steer this collective feeling in the direction of political action, but morale, and beneath it *esprit de corps*, prime agents, collectively, for such action. Both identity and morale belong to my category of 'discourse'.

Blumer emphasises that there is nothing necessary about the emergence of the various cultural elements he describes or about any effects they may have. However, he claims that *esprit de corps*, morale and ideology each provide a soil out of which more formal organisation may grow. They are elementary forms of human organisation. Moreover, he argues that they may be further enhanced through the emergence of more formal organisational mechanisms. In this respect his account focuses upon both diffuse movement currents and what I, following Zald and McCarthy (1994), have called SMOs. For a diffuse current to fully become a movement, he appears to claim, presupposes the (contingent) emergence of organisational forms and thus SMOs, which, as the wording suggests, constitute its organisational nuclei. Furthermore, he effectively offers an account of the birth of SMOs which views them as an organic outgrowth of the emergence of movements and cultures of contention.

So far I have spoken primarily of the formation of discourse. I have said little of its spread beyond noting the diffusion role taken up by many SMOs. I hope it is evident, however, that discourses, because social (i.e. collective) phenomena, already have some degree of 'spread'. Discourses take shape, as noted above, within and as an effect of the interactions of a group, such that they are always already spread through the group. It should also be evident that collective action is dependent upon further diffusion. Collective action will only spread through the population or achieve wider support to the extent that relevant discourses are likewise diffused, whether deliberately, by SMOs, or unintentionally in the course of everyday interaction and the work of the mass media.

## Precipitating factors

Precipitating factors are trigger events which provide an impetus and concrete focus for mobilisation. The police beating of Rodney King and subsequent acquittal of the officers involved, which triggered the LA riots of 1992, is one example of this. Another is Rosa Parks's ejection from a bus for refusing to give her seat over to a white man, in 1955, which triggered the Montgomery bus boycott and played a central role in the wider mobilisation of the US black civil rights movement. Precipitating factors are important because strains can sometimes be quite abstract and have a long history, making it difficult both to mobilise populations around them and to raise claims about them in public contexts. Mobilisation requires something more tangible to latch on to; a discrete event which exemplifies wider strains and has the power to shock, generating sympathy and thus adherents and constituents.

The effect of such events may be purely spontaneous and may, as the name suggests, both precipitate and trigger significant SMO/movement developments. Key actors may become involved in struggle only after and as an effect of them. Equally, however, precipitating factors can be selected by SMOs. It is well known, for example, that Rosa Parks's ejection from the bus in Montgomery was not the first event of its kind. She was a civil rights activist, an active member of an SMO, and her particular ejection was selected as a trigger event because she, in contrast to many who had earlier done what she did, was a woman of 'good character' who could better symbolise the injustice of American racism than others who had refused to give up their seat, and whose life could not withstand the scrutiny it was bound to attract. In addition, much of the framing work of SMOs is focused upon events which, if interpreted 'appropriately', could trigger wider mobilisation. Note also that selection may be retroactive. Events of the past can be rediscovered, re-ignited and re-interpreted for mobilisation purposes, either because agitators are looking for them or because a discursive shift casts them in a fresh light.

## Mobilisation of participants for action

This involves the organisational and communicative structures which facilitate mobilisation. The process of mobilisation, Smelser argues, requires that agents are capable of coordinating themselves and this, in turn, presupposes: effective communication channels, perhaps a chain of command and often a division of labour. In making this point Smelser anticipates much that has been written more recently on the topic of networks and social movements (e.g. Diani and McAdam 2003, Gould 1991, Snow *et al.* 1980, Tilly 1978). Much movement research suggests that it is often pre-existing groups and networks who mobilise for action rather than individuals, particularly groups whose members share a salient identity (Tilly 1978). Likewise, it is suggested that pre-existing groups fare-better in struggle (Gould 1991). The obvious example of this is the black civil rights movement in the United States, which grew out of a network of black churches and colleges (McAdam 1982, Morris 1984). It was not individuals who mobilised in this context but rather congregations and student bodies. Furthermore, many of the early leaders of the civil rights movements, the obvious example being the Reverend Martin Luther King, were religious leaders in their communities. They led their community in political opposition as they led them in prayer, and their availability for leadership was a crucial factor in mobilisation. The reason why it is often pre-existing networks who mobilise, rather than isolated individuals, is, first, that bringing together isolated individuals into any form of coordinated whole is an enormous and resource-intensive task, even when only small numbers are involved, such that mobilisation is more likely when collectivisation has already been achieved. Second, to reiterate, already existing groups have the channels of communication, organisation, leadership and so on necessary for effective mobilisation. Indeed, already existing groups may 'possess' a whole range of important resources which, by definition, an aggregate of unconnected individuals could not possess: for example, mutual trust, *esprit de corps*, collective identity, rapport, mutual support mechanisms, shared situational definitions and so on.

Smelser's argument is also quite close to that of Zald and McCarthy, discussed in Chapter 1. Although he doesn't use the concept of SMOs or draw a distinction between movements and organisation he, like Blumer (see above), appears to be saying that *organisational forms are necessary if sentiments (beliefs and demands) are to be translated into action*. The way each develops this point is different. Blumer, as noted, claims that organisational forms emerge (or don't) organically in the course of the interactions which constitute emergent cultures of contention, whereas Smelser focuses upon pre-existing organisational arrangements (which may or may not be in place) and Zald and McCarthy look to political entrepreneurs who 'play' political markets, responding to and cultivating political demand in the pursuit of rewards (see Chapter 1). The underlying recognition of the significance of organisation and organisations (SMOs) is a constant factor in all three theories, however. SMOs are contingent developments in contentious situations but where they do emerge, they have a significant impact.

For my part I cannot see why we have to assume that all SMOs emerge in the same way. Different SMOs may emerge by different paths; sometimes organically, sometimes out of pre-existing organisational forms, other times though the effort of political entrepreneurs. We see examples of each of these paths in the analysis of the later chapters. By whatever path they emerge, however, the birth of SMOs within a movement or contentious context is important because the organisation that is definitive of them, and that, as I have said, may bear no resemblance to the 'economically rational' organisation assumed by Zald and McCarthy (see Chapter 1), transforms vague demands and sentiments into actions.

### Operation of social control

The final factor that Smelser discusses is the impact of the reaction of agencies of social control, amongst whom he includes the state, the police and the media. Agencies of social control can sometimes prevent or quell movement formation, either by mollifying agitated populations or by sheer force and repression. By the same token they can accelerate and amplify movement formation by, for example, launching an ineffective and (in the eyes of the wider population) illegitimate attempt to control a movement. It is not uncommon in the history of movements for a televised confrontation between protestors and police, in which the latter seem heavy-handed, to provoke further mobilisation.

Smelser treats the media as an agency of social control in this context. I prefer to think of the media as a field in which struggles may be (partly) conducted, and which may or may not be structurally conducive for such struggles, as discussed earlier. The journalists, editors, film makers and others who populate this field are agents. But they are not necessarily agents of social control. As I have noted in research on 'anti-corporate' struggles, some journalists are also activists and can combine their journalistic and activist roles, using their access to the means of publicity to great effect (Crossley 2002b). Furthermore, many journalists are looking for a good story, something which will satisfy the demands of their editor, and they will run the story in whatever way best works to suit their own needs and wants. The media field is a 'game' with its own rules and imperatives, which does not automatically fulfil given political functions and which enjoys at least a certain degree of autonomy from the immediate wants of the power elite. I do not deny that the media world, tied as it is so often is to rich media magnates and advertisers, is free of elite influence. There is a distinct game of journalism and journalistic integrity, however, which both inspires certain journalists to push at the boundaries of the *status quo*, questioning the legitimacy of established elites and their decisions, and which filters political influence. Moreover, there are norms of good journalistic practice which journalists and editors are expected and pressured to adhere to, wherever this may 'lead'. I believe that the media is better considered as a field composed of actors whose views and actions can be quite diverse. There are radical journalists and editors, sympathetic to social movements, who operate outside of the conventional boundaries of politics. There are more conservative journalists and editors who are unsympathetic. And there are many besides: to the left, the right, the centre, populists, libertarians, authoritarians and others. These camps jostle alongside one another and alongside proprietors, advertisers and others. Their individual output is shaped by these relations and interactions.

This is true also of solicitors and the legal game, politicians and the parliamentary game, and perhaps even police officers and the policing game, though the policing 'game' is a game of social control and so will tend to reflect more directly the social control imperative. Each of these 'agencies' is in fact a diverse field with its own imperatives, rules, stakes and dynamics. The agents involved in these fields will very often become 'third parties' to political contention but their interventions will seldom be reducible to a one-dimensional control function. Their engagement will be shaped by the significance which the specific contention, protest or movement enjoys within their own field. Struggle can be an opportunity for civil rights lawyers, for example, or indeed for aspiring politicians in opposition parties seeking evidence of public dissatisfaction and government mismanagement. And their efforts to exploit it may be of direct benefit to the movement involved. Whilst Smelser is right to note the significance of *third parties*, therefore, he is wrong to reduce their intervention to *the function of social control*. I will refer to *third parties* rather than social control in my model – although I include agencies who may act in controlling ways within this notion of third parties.

It will be remembered from the previous chapter that third parties are also an important element in the concept of fields of contention. In Chapter 1 I discussed this in terms of the role of third parties in relations of structural equivalence. The present discussion, however, has hopefully given a clearer sense of the importance of interactions between activists/SMOs and third parties in their own right. It is also important, in this connection, to note the generative dynamics that can take shape in interactions between protest groups and third parties. McAdam (1983) provides an excellent example of this in his account of the interactions between police and protestors in the context of the black civil rights movement. He notes that initial activities by the protestors caught the authorities off guard. They were innovative and the authorities were not sure how to respond. For this reason, the protests were successful, and their success generated further support for the movement amongst its potential constituent population. Success boosted recruitment. Over time, however, the authorities were able to take stock and devise policing strategies which effectively contained and controlled the protestors. Consequently protests became less effective, and this had a negative effect upon levels of support and recruitment. That is, until the protestors thought up new tactics, which again caught the authorities off guard, were successful and boosted support etc. McAdam likens this situation to a game of chess, with each party trying to outwit the other and proving highly innovative in the process. The action of each party was a reaction to the action of the others, such that the parties constituted an interaction system with its own irreducible dynamics and trajectory. This is, of course, exactly the argument I have made with respect to the interactions between SMOs which constitute fields of contention and is the key reason for including third parties in our definition of these fields. They too belong to the irreducible dynamic of interaction constitutive of a field. Moreover, note that this irreducible interaction system drew innovation and imagination out of its participants. In finding solutions to the obstacles posed by the other each party, to some extent, had to reinvent the art of protest.

The qualification, 'to some extent', is important. Reflecting upon protest over centuries, Charles Tilly (1977, 1978, 1986, 1995) has argued that specific time–spaces tend to have relatively stable repertoires of protest techniques which are drawn upon time and again: what he calls 'repertoires of contention' (for elaboration and critique see also Traugott 1995 etc., Crossley 2002a). Agents choose how to protest, Tilly (1995) argues, but they do so on the basis of the options they have learned; options which, at any point of time, are 'limited'. Different agents in different struggles draw upon the same repertoire. Having said this, Tilly notes that the techniques that comprise a repertoire at any point have been forged by innovative agents engaged in struggle, and he adds that repertoires change, adding new and dropping old techniques, as an effect of struggle.

## Restating the position

In the above discussion, drawing upon more recent movement theory and analysis, I have attempted to modernise the six basic elements of Smelser's model. My new list is as follows:

1 Structural conduciveness (including both resource flows/availability and various 'opportunity structures').
2 Structural strain, understood as a mismatch between expectations and reality.
3 Discursive formation and diffusion (which includes frames, theories, ideologies, narratives of collective self-understanding and identity).
4 Trigger events.
5 Mobilising structures (including organisational forms and, most centrally, SMOs).
6 Intervention of third parties.

In each case, moreover, I have attempted to fit the model more closely to my conception of movements, SMOs and fields, as defined in Chapter 1 (see also below). In particular, I have argued that strain and discursive formation/ diffusion correspond to movement formation, with mobilising structures and organisational forms being necessary for the additional development of SMOs. I have also suggested that the intervention of third parties corresponds to what I said about third parties in my discussion of fields. Having re-defined these basic categories, however, I follow Smelser to the letter in insisting both that they are analytic, such that the same event, condition etc. might register twice on the model, and that the order in which they come into play will vary across cases. In some cases, new social strains lead almost immediately to protest because the other conditions are already adequately met. In other cases, strains may have no noticeable political effect for years because the discourses and mobilising structures necessary to translate them into action are missing, or perhaps because conditions are not conducive: for example, resources are lacking or political control repressive. Likewise a shift in political opportunities can precipitate new struggles. Even trigger-events can precede the protests they trigger by many years, if, for example, they are rediscovered and re-energised as a consequence of new discursive formations.

Before concluding this chapter I want to say a brief word further about fields. The value-added model really speaks more to the emergence of movements and SMOs than to fields. However, in doing so it does effectively describes the origins of fields. The conditions that give rise to one movement or SMO can very easily and more likely give rise to more than one. The same conditions will spawn more than one SMO and possibly more than one movement. These SMOs will, of necessity, initiate interactions with the same third parties and therefore, at the very least, find themselves in relations of structural equivalence. Moreover, this in turn will tend to generate situations in which their members meet (e.g. at demonstrations, meetings etc.), leading to the emergence of relationships between them. In short, a field will take shape.

## Conclusion

The purpose of this chapter has been to outline a theoretical model of the emrgence of social movements, SMOs and fields of contention. The model was based upon the value-added model of Neil Smelser which, I argued, is problematic but also useful and interesting. In Chapters 4–7, I put this theoretical framework into action. First, however, it is necessary to briefly consider the historical background context of contemporary psychiatric politics. That is the task of Chapter 3.

# 3   Contextualising contention
## A potted history of the mental health field

In this chapter I offer a schematic outline of the history of psychiatry in the United Kingdom. This serves three purposes. First, it describes the context in which UK mental health politics has emerged, allowing us to identify some of the strains, opportunities and constraints that have shaped it. Second, as a long-term historical survey, it allows us to avoid the myopia that can result from too narrow a temporal frame. The earlier history of psychiatry affords us a point of comparison against which to gauge its more recent political history. Third, it allows us to see that the history of psychiatry is a history of struggle and contention whilst simultaneously laying a foundation that will allow us, later in the book, to appreciate what is novel about contemporary struggles. For reasons of space my account will be brief, schematic and descriptive. I will only be discussing those aspects of psychiatry that I deem necessary to fulfil the three purposes outlined above and only in a 'scene setting' manner. The account is adequate to its purposes, however.

## The beginning

Medical models of madness can be traced back, in the history of West, to the ancient Greeks. Although the ancients did not make the same distinction that we make between 'mental' and 'physical' life, we can find disease categories in the works of such writers as Hippocrates and Galen which incorporate forms of what we now call 'mental illness' (Porter 2002). And these writers claimed that such illnesses had organic causes which could be treated medically (ibid.). The later emergence of Christianity obscured this picture by introducing the notion of an immortal soul and various alternative interpretations of madness but the rediscovery and translation of central Greek texts during the Renaissance ensured a continued influence of these texts, at least until the late seventeenth century (ibid.).

It would be a mistake to infer from this, however, that psychiatry or a mental health field existed before the end of the seventeenth century. Medicine was largely undifferentiated before this time. All doctors tended to treat most illnesses, with very few specialists. There was, in the UK, a rudimentary division between 'barber surgeons', who had received a royal charter in 1462, 'physicians', who won their royal charter in 1518, and 'apothecaries',[1] who were granted the right to monopolise the practice of dispensing drugs in London in 1617 (Busfield 1986). The division of medicine into the specialised branches we are familiar with today had not yet occurred, however, and with the exception of a handful of cases, there was no specialisation around the treatment of the mad until the early eighteenth century (Busfield 1986, Porter 1987a). More importantly, with one exception there were no specialised sites for the control, containment or treatment of madness. The exception was the Priory of the Order of St Mary of Bethlehem ('Bethlem' or 'Bedlam'), which was founded in London in 1247 and first used to house lunatics in 1377. This is an exception, however, as the second public madhouse in the United Kingdom, Bethal in Northwhich, was not opened until 1713, and there is very little evidence of private madhouses existing before 1600. This is significant because the madhouses were the locus around which psychiatry took shape.

## Private madhouses

Although very little is known about the earliest of these houses, it is likely that they grew out of lodging arrangements for single individuals (Porter 1987a). Certainly the earliest known examples catered at most for a handful of inmates. As there was no requirement for these houses to be registered, prior to 1774, it is not possible to gauge the numbers of such houses in the early eighteenth century. Records indicate that there were 16 in London by 1774, however, and this figure had risen to 40 by 1819. In the provinces there were 22 registered houses in 1802, and that figure had risen to 49 by 1819 (ibid.). The national total, according to Scull's (1993) figures, rose from 45 to 139 between 1807 and 1844. Moreover, the size of these houses was increasing too. Though many were small, some were catering for between 100 and 500 inmates by the mid-nineteenth century.

There are varied accounts of why these houses began to emerge. Mechanic (1969) suggests that the changes associated with industrialisation (e.g. increased geographical mobility, new urban living arrangements and population increase) made it more difficult for families to care for their own mentally disturbed members, thereby generating a demand for provision to which bourgeois entrepreneurs responded. Scull (1993) disputes this, however, noting both that the growth of private madhouses pre-dates the main thrust of industrialisation in Britain and that the location of these houses does not match with the geography of early industrial development. A more likely explanation, Scull argues, is that the breakdown of the feudal order and the emergence of capitalist social relations destroyed the traditional social structures that made it possible for families to care for their dependent members. Some of these unproductive members could be directed to the workhouses and poorhouses which were beginning to develop in the eighteenth century but, Scull argues, this was not true of the mad whose antics tended to exclude them. The mad caused havoc in workhouses, he notes, generating a demand for alternatives. He quotes a document from St Lukes Hospital, from 1750, which illustrates the basic point:

> The law has made no particular provision for lunatiks and it must be allowed that the common parish workhouse (the inhabitants of which are mostly aged and infirm people) are very unfit places for the reception of such ungovernable and mischievous persons, who necessarily require separate apartments.
>
> (cited in Scull 1993, 39)

Not that the problem was solved instantly. A report from 1807 states that

> The number of other Pauper Lunatics in Poor Houses and Houses of Industry, according to the returns received, amounts to 1,765, exclusive of 483 in private custody; but these are so evidently deficient in several instances, that a large addition must be made in any computation of the whole number.
>
> (House of Commons, *Report of the Select Committee on the State of the Criminal and Pauper Lunatics*, 1807)

It goes on to claim that the mad caused confusion and chaos in such confined spaces. Thus there was a perceived need for a different place to contain the mad.

Scull's account would lead us to predict that the inmates of the madhouses were primarily working class, if not paupers, and that the houses themselves would be akin to the workhouses which otherwise serviced the working class. This is true of some madhouses but not all of them. A significant proportion of madhouse inmates were middle class and some madhouses were designed specifically to appeal to this economic class. A further explanation of 'the trade in lunacy', offered by Roy Porter (1987a), speaks more to this client base. The eighteenth century was a time of economic growth, affluence and the emergence of a service sector in England, Porter argues. Britain was becoming a 'consumer society' (see also Porter 1982). Private madhouses were a part of this growing service boom:

> Madhouses and mad-doctors arose from the same soil which generated demand for general practitioners, dancing masters, man midwives, face painters, drawing tutors, estate managers, landscape gardeners, architects, journalists and that host of other white collar, service and quasi-professional occupations which a society with increased economic surplus and pretensions to civilisation first found it could afford, and soon found it could not do without. In the 'birth of the consumer society', one growing item of consumption was the services of madhouses, not

because affluence drove people crazy, but because its commercial ethos made trading in insanity feasible.

(Porter 1987a, 165)

Porter supports this argument by pointing to the initially slow uptake of certain madhouses and the considerable efforts that their owners went to, to drum up trade (see also Busfield 1986). The emergence of madhouses was not an entrepreneurial response to an urgent demand, from this point of view, but rather 'supply led':

> When Ticehurst was founded, custom was initially a mere trickle, indicating that demand had to be 'created' or at least nursed, rather than being a damned-up lake seeking outlet. Nevertheless, once a 'supply' was created, demand soon rose to capacity.
>
> (Porter 1987a, 165)

There was no requirement in the early days of the madhouses that medics be involved in them and many were free of medical intervention. However, as Porter notes, there were considerable incentives on the part of medics to become involved. The growth of the medical profession was generating an increased pressure for specialisation within it; mad doctoring was one such path of specialisation. In addition, madhouses were lucrative because one could charge for bed and board as well as for medical treatment. Many medics made a fortune out of private madhouses (ibid.). It is perhaps for these reasons that, in time, medics began to stake out a claim to monopoly in relation to madhouses and the 'treatment' of madness. Madness and its care, they began to assert, were their domain. And they were prepared to campaign to secure their claim.

## Lunacy reform

The battle for medical monopoly was not the only struggle taking shape around the madhouses in the eighteenth century, however. At the same time, a movement of 'lunacy reform' was emerging. Initially, this movement focused upon wrongful confinement in madhouses. Later in its history, however, it challenged the treatment to which inmates of the madhouses were subject (Busfield 1986, Scull 1989, 1993). It was common in many madhouses, for example, for inmates to be manacled to the walls of freezing cold cells, without any source of heat or sanitation. And it was not uncommon for madhouse owners to 'tame' their inmates with a whip. Indeed, some boasted in pamphlets of their abilities with the whip (ibid.).

The reason that madhouse keepers felt able to boast of their ability with the whip and kept their inmates in freezing cold cells, according to Scull (1989), was that the mad were deemed by many to be animals, and animals were deemed insensitive to pain and cold. Although there were various competing social representations of madness at the time, this popular and sometimes dominant representation lent legitimacy to harsh treatment, and even recommended it. By the same token, the reason that these practices became subject to critique and calls for reform is that representations, during the period of the Enlightenment, were changing. Enlightenment discourse encouraged questioning and critique of previously taken-for-granted practices, beliefs and representations. Common sense and popular prejudice were overturned. In addition, moral sensibilities and categories were changing. More specifically, however, new conceptions of both the nervous system and the role of learning in human development were generating a new conception of madness. It came to be viewed as the result of faulty learning. No longer viewed as animals, the mad came to be seen as children in need of moral guidance and a good upbringing. In itself this provided good reason to be critical of the conditions and harsh treatment of the madhouses, particularly as new Enlightenment representations of children encouraged a caring, nurturing attitude. In addition, however, new understandings of madness gave rise to new, high profile techniques of treatment which were perceived to be highly effective. Enthusiasm for and belief in this new form of treatment fuelled further critique of the whips and manacles regime.

A famous illustration of this new 'moral treatment', as it was called, is that of George III. After his own doctors failed to help him, the king was treated by Francis Willis, a renowned advocate of moral treatment (MacAlpine and Hunter 1993). Like many advocates of moral treatment, Willis believed that whips were not necessary to control the mad and that 'capturing the eye' (i.e. a stern look and eye-to-eye contact) was quite sufficient. In addition, he used a system of rewards and punishments and he communicated trust to the king, generating a moral pressure to behave. Reward, punishment, trust and the eye were the basis of moral treatment. And George III was a very high profile success story for the approach, or so it seemed (ibid.).

Besides the treatment of the king, the other key focus for many advocates of moral treatment, particularly in the early nineteenth century, was the York Retreat, opened in 1796 by the Quaker, William Tuke, following the mysterious death of a fellow Quaker at the York Asylum in 1790, and the reluctance of the Asylum's custodians to shed any light upon this death (Digby 1985a,b). The Retreat, which initially relied entirely upon moral treatment and eschewed any form of medical intervention, was highly successful. It became a shining example of good practice and a key reference point for lunacy reformers throughout Europe. Many believed that, with the Retreat, they had found a way forward for the treatment of 'lunatiks' and the reputation of the institution quickly grew strong.

The origin of lunacy reform dates back at least as far as 1763, when a series of scandals involving both cruelty and wrongful confinement prompted a parliamentary committee. The committee recommended reform but legislation was delayed by eleven years because of opposition by the

Royal College of Physicians. When finally passed, the 1774 *Act for Regulating Private Madhouses* required licencing of all private madhouses; the keeping of registers; medical certification for all lunatics kept in mad-houses, except pauper lunatics; and a system of inspection of madhouses, which in London was to be organised by the Royal College (magistrates were charged with this responsibility in the provinces). The impetus for change died down after this report. It was to pick up again in the early nineteenth century, however, until the middle of that century. The efforts of campaigners prompted a series of parliamentary reports and acts (see Table 3.1), which effectively laid the ground for a mid-century shift in mental health provision, from a private to a public system.

The reformers were drawn from two main sources (Scull 1993). Some were magistrates who were often involved in the inspection of madhouses and were familiar with the range of problems being thrown up by the social changes characteristic of this period. Others were drawn from a ready-made camp of bourgeois reformers and philanthropists who were active in relation to a range of issues. Activists from within these two camps were, in turn, motivated by one of two ideological stances: reactionary Christian evangelism and Benthamite utilitarianism. Whereas the Christians were largely concerned to recover what they believed was a lost morality and to rescue the poor from vice, degradation and moral decline, the Benthamites were looking forward, seeking to maximise the cultural advances of the Enlightenment by instituting a rational approach to governance and administration. The

*Table 3.1* Lunacy reform in the nineteenth century

| | |
|---|---|
| 1807 | A parliamentary select committee investigates provision in a number of madhouses, as well as instances where lunatics have been kept in poorhouses. It recommends provision of public asylums |
| 1808 | *The Lunatics Act* authorises (but does not compel) counties and boroughs to build and run asylums using public money |
| 1815/16 | A parliamentary select committee is set up following scandals at both Bethlehem and the York Asylum |
| 1827 | A further select committee on 'metropolitan madhouses' is called |
| 1828 | *The Madhouses Act* improves inspection at metropolitan madhouses Metropolitan lunacy commissioners assume responsibility for licencing and inspection |
| 1829 | *The County Asylums Act* requires county asylums to provide details of all admissions, discharges and deaths to the home office |
| 1845 | *The Lunatics Act* establishes a permanent national Lunacy Commission (with a strong medical representation on it) and requires that all asylums keep a medical visitation and a record of all medical treatments administered |
| 1845 | *The Lunatic Asylums Act* compels all county and borough authorities to erect public asylums |
| 1890 | *The Lunacy Act* tightens procedures for admission and certification, extending and further securing the role of both medical and legal professionals |

horrors of the madhouses, for this latter group, were a sign of an amateurish approach to administration. The situation needed to be systematised and rationalised by way of a strict regime of inspection, record keeping etc.

In an interesting twist the Benthamites, whom one would ordinarily associate with free market liberalism, were strong advocates of a public system of madhouse provision. The drive to cut costs and maximise profits was a key cause of malpractice and problems in their view. All camps of reformers, moreover, were inspired by the York Retreat. It was their model of good practice and their proof both that madness could be cured and that better alternatives were possible.

Those on the receiving end of psychiatry had little involvement in this movement, except in a few instances where 'alleged lunatics' gave evidence to parliamentary committees, usually in relation to issues of wrongful confinement. Some of those on the receiving end published pamphlets, however, criticising the treatment to which they were subject, making their own calls for reform and often protesting their sanity (Porter 1987b). The main examples are

- Samuel Bruckshaw (1774) *The Case, Petition and Address of Samuel Bruckshaw, who suffered a most severe imprisonment for almost a year.*
- Samuel Bruckshaw (1774) *One More Proof of the Iniquitous Abuse of Private Madhouses.*
- William Belcher (1796) *Address to Humanity, Containing a Letter to Dr Monro, a Receipt to Make a Lunatic and a Sketch of a True Smiling Hyena.*
- John Perceval (1838 and 1840) *A Narrative of the Treatment Received by a Gentleman, During a State of Mental Derangement* (two volumes).
- Richard Paternoster (1841) *The Madhouse System.*

The authors of these pamphlets were not average madhouse inmates. They were literate, well connected and well resourced. John Perceval, as the son of the assassinated Prime Minister, Spencer Perceval, is only the most obvious example of this. Perceval is also important, moreover, since he was behind the earliest documented collective of 'alleged lunatics' in the historical record, the 'Alleged Lunatics' Friend Society' (ALFS) (Hervey 1986, Hunter and MacAlpine 1961). The ALFS were quite unlike any of the 'survivor' SMOs that I will be considering in this book and, as far as I can tell, are the only known group for 'alleged lunatics' to emerge in the nineteenth century. Their existence is interesting, however, even if somewhat anomalous.

How seriously these 'lunatiks' accounts were taken is not clear from the historical record. There is evidence that some accounts were more or less dismissed because their authors were deemed mad and thus unreliable. Indeed, we find evidence of this kind of reception as late as the 1950s (see Chapter 4). Even the eminently rational lunacy reformers encountered fierce opposition, however. A public sphere took shape with advocates of a variety of positions thrashing out their differences. Referring to a parliamentary inquiry of 1815/16, for example, Scull notes that

> A furious press and pamphlet war took place during the whole of this time, keeping the case continuously before the public, and providing a highly effective forum for the dissemination of the reformers ideas to an ever wider audience.
>
> (Scull 1993, 111)

In opposition to the reformers were both madhouse keepers and medics. Madhouse keepers resisted for the obvious reason that they did not like being criticised and did not want to have to pay for the reforms being proposed. Medics resisted because they too were a focus of criticism and because the high profile and apparent success of moral treatment cast doubt upon their own less effective approach. Medics were part of the problem, as far as the lunacy reformers were concerned. And they became part of the resistance.

By the mid-nineteenth century, however, many medics had changed strategy (Porter 1987a). They became advocates of moral treatment. They were careful to point out, however, that the mad often also suffered from physical and organic problems, such that a simultaneously physical and moral approach to madness was necessary. They were, of course, in the best position to offer this, given their expertise on the physical side. Making this argument stick was an important step in their eventual success at securing a monopoly on the treatment of lunacy.

Repeatedly the lunacy reformers won the argument regarding the need for a public asylum system. The reality was only achieved in stages, however. The *Lunatics Act* of 1808 authorised county and borough authorities to use public money to build asylums. But very few did. It was not until the *Lunatic Asylums Act* of 1845 that public asylum provision became mandatory.

## The nineteenth century asylum system

Although development was uneven and some counties initially resisted (Scull 1993), the 1845 legislation paved the way for a massive increase in the numbers of asylums. In 1827, there were only 9 county borough or city asylums. This had jumped to 24 by 1850, immediately after the 1845 legislation. And by 1930 the figure was 98. A national system of public asylums was emerging (Figure 3.1). In this respect the dream of the lunacy reformers was beginning to be realised. In other, crucial respects, however, the plans of the lunacy reformers were compromised. One of the main arguments against the asylums had been their cost and when they were introduced considerations of cost quickly overrode the reformers' ideals. At one level, this involved compromises regarding decoration. The reformers had wanted

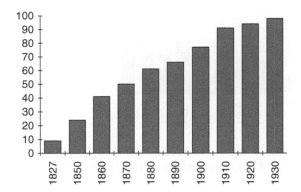

*Figure 3.1* Number of county borough asylums in Britain 1827–1930.

Source: Jones, K. (1972) *A History of the Mental Health Services*, London, RKP.

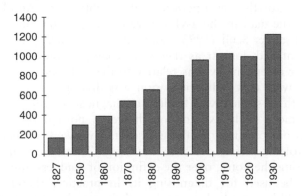

*Figure 3.2* Average number of patients in county asylums in Britain 1827–1930.

Source: Jones, K. (1972) *A History of the Mental Health Services*, London, RKP.

public asylums to embody a homely, family atmosphere, as at the York Retreat. This didn't happen. Asylums were furnished in a drab, minimalist fashion, with very little to make them seem homely. More importantly, however, the size of asylums was considerably increased, to a point where any hope of moral treatment or a family atmosphere was obliterated. In 1827, the average number of inmates in any public asylum was 166. By 1930 this figure had increased to 1221 (Figure 3.2).

Moreover, as the number and size of asylums grew, so did the relative proportion of the general population officially diagnosed as insane (Figure 3.3). Indeed, rates of insanity were growing so rapidly that two special Parliamentary reports were commissioned to look into and assess the problem (Scull 1993). A number of different explanations were offered.

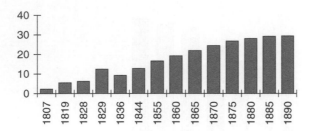

*Figure 3.3* Rates of insanity per 10,000 of the population 1807–90.

Source: Scull, A. (1993) *The Most Solitary of Afflictions*, New Haven, Yale University Press.

In the first instance, it was suggested that rising figures of insanity represented a backlog. This would only account for an initial surge, however, not for sustained growth over a period of over eighty years. Another explanation was that the mad in the asylums were living longer, but this still doesn't make sense. As Scull (1993) notes, life expectancies weren't changing to that extent and, insofar as they were changing, they weren't improving to a greater extent in asylums relative to the wider population. Two further theories were that industrialisation was driving people mad and/or that the growth of science was leading to diagnosis of previously undetected cases. A more likely explanation, however, posited by Scull (1993), is that definitions of lunacy at the grassroots level were widening and thresholds of tolerance for deviance lowering. There was much disagreement at this time, he notes, over the definition of madness and the criteria that should be used for diagnosing it. In practice, therefore, diagnostic criteria could be stretched or condensed in accordance with the availability of treatment facilities. He suggests three reasons why the boundaries might have been stretched. First, humanitarian motives made the asylum doctors predisposed towards a wider rather than a narrower definition of madness. Like any other doctor, they tended, in unclear cases, to assume that treatment is required in order to avoid leaving sick patients untreated. Second, it was in the professional interests of the doctors to define madness as widespread. The bigger the problem, the more money and status would be attached to those who had to deal with it. The explanation can't rest entirely at the door of the professionals, according to Scull, however. His third argument is that the existence of the asylum lowered the tolerance thresholds of the community, with respect to unusual behaviour, generating a demand for sequestration: 'If we make a convenient lumber room, we all know how speedily it becomes filled with lumber. The county asylum is the mental lumber room of the surrounding district' (Scull 1993, 373).

There are two indicators within the trends which Scull cites as evidence for this interpretation. First, he notes that his thesis would lead one to expect that the number of pauper lunatics would rise more sharply than better-off lunatics because pauper lunatics were less able to escape the judgements of the community. This expectation is confirmed. The rise in numbers of lunatics was overwhelmingly amongst paupers. Second, he argues that one would expect the shift to be 'supply led'; that is, one would expect estimates of insanity to go up as facilities increase. This too is confirmed.

It is not just the presence of the asylums that explains this reduction in the level of community tolerance, however. Industrialisation put strain upon families and communities, reducing their capacity to care for their dependent members. And the 1834 Poor Law Amendment Act abolished outdoor relief, tying relief to confinement in either a workhouse or asylum. This made unproductive individuals a financial burden upon their families and created an incentive to have them incarcerated. Moreover, as Busfield (1986) points out, the shift in work locations, from the home to the factory, made practical care at home impossible.

## Custodialism

Asylums were custodial institutions. It is clear, for example, that great emphasis was put upon security within them and very little upon comfort. High walls, closed doors and tight security measures shut them off from the outside, whereas inside physical restraint was often used. Moreover, research suggests that very little treatment went on in practice. Internal population sizes prevented the possibility of any moral treatment and it is well documented that the medics involved in the asylum became little more than administrators of it (Busfield 1986). They seldom attended patients and when they did it was more likely for physical problems unrelated to insanity. Stays tended to be lengthy and even official cure rates were very low.

This custodial character did not pass unnoticed at the time, either amongst medics or the public. There was a public critique of the asylum running right through the latter part of the nineteenth century. Henry Maudsley, for example, who founded the Maudsley Hospital, denied that asylums were in any sense hospitals and described them as '...vast receptacles for the concealment and safekeeping of lunacy' (cited in Busfield 1986, 265). Such arguments were accompanied, moreover, by continued attempts to implement changes. It was to be a long time, however, before any significant change took place to alter this situation.

The growing population sizes inside the asylums contributed to the development and maintenance of their custodial characteristics. Asylums which had originally been intended for 300 or so inmates were now required to hold over 1000 and, as a consequence, were able to do little more than contain. As Busfield has argued, however, the connection of the asylum system to that of the poor law was at least as significant. She argues that the Poor Law:

> ...affected the numbers, flow and characteristics of the inmates to be found in them; it affected the scale and size of institutions; it affected the resources available to them including the numbers, qualifications and attitudes of the medical men and the attendants who worked within them; and it affected the responses to policy initiatives to improve and reform them.
>
> (Busfield 1986, 266)

Moreover, it established the asylum as a place of last resort and made it function as a deterrent. Certification was a lengthy and difficult process and the conditions inside the asylum were generally unpleasant. This prevented the asylum from becoming an attractive alternative to either the workhouse or work itself and, in Busfield's view, this was intentional.

At the same time as the asylums were growing, the psychiatric profession was beginning to establish itself more formally. One of the early steps in this process was the formation, in 1841, of the Association of Medical Officers of Asylums and Hospitals for the Insane. This professional association was weak at first because it had no journal. The only forum for interaction and exchange between its members was a yearly conference. Consequently there was little coordination or solidarity among them. This situation was amended in 1853, when the association founded the *Asylum Journal*. By this time, however, another journal devoted exclusively to the medicine of the mind had already been launched: the *Journal of Psychological Medicine and Mental Pathology*. The profession was growing and strengthening.

In both journals, as well as a variety of pamphlets, increasing emphasis was placed on the physical basis of madness. Lunacy was increasingly viewed, contrary to earlier claims about moral treatment, as an organically rooted illness which required proper, medical treatment. Insofar as treatments were administered within the asylum, which, as noted earlier, was rarely, they tended to be physical treatments: for example, emetics, purgatives, opium, hot and cold baths. By way of these claims, the medical profession was able to extend its claim for a monopoly on psychiatric treatment. It was argued that the treatment of insanity required the skills of the medically trained. Moreover, the asylum system furthered the possibility for specialisation by establishing an apprenticeship system; newly qualified doctors could take up a junior position at an asylum and learn their trade.

There was a problem, however. Although medicine was making advances elsewhere, psychiatric treatments were not very effective. There were no big breakthroughs, as in other areas of medicine, and the cure rate, as noted above, was very low. This was recognised, at least in respect of chronic patients, by the profession itself. A number of reports and manuals of the 1850s note the ineffectiveness of existing physical treatments and suggest that they either make no difference or exacerbate problems. By this time, however, the medical model was deeply entrenched and thus the basic assumption of physical causation was not open to question.

## The twentieth century

The psychiatric field has been transformed quite considerably in the course of the twentieth century. Busfield (1986) points out four main points of transformation. First, it has shifted away from a largely homogeneous form of provision, centred upon the asylum, towards a heterogeneous ensemble of forms of provision located at a variety of sites within the community: for example, home treatment, outpatient clinics, day centres etc. Second, there has been a massive increase in numbers of people receiving help for what are medically defined as psychiatric problems. For the first part of the century this meant an increase in asylum numbers, as we saw above, but since the 1950s it has meant increases in outpatients and in people seeing their General Practitioners (GPs). Third, this has involved a shift in the balance of problems dealt with by psychiatric services, particularly in the public sector, as much of the growth in diagnosis and treatment has centred upon the previously marginal neurotic and personality disorders. Moreover we might add here, that psychiatry and the wider 'psy' disciplines have increasingly adopted a proactive stance in the latter part of the twentieth century, seeking to manage and promote 'mental health' across a variety of everyday contexts (Miller and Rose 1988, Rose 1985, 1988, 1989, 1992). Finally, there has been a shift in the social character of patients. On the one hand the average age of psychiatric patients tends to be older now, as psychiatrists have begun to examine problems which are more common in the elderly (e.g. Alzheimer's disease). On the other hand, psychiatry now treats far more women and middle class people than in the past (Busfield 1996, Showalter 1987). The 1930 *Mental Treatment Act* and the events leading up to it constitute a useful focal point for making sense of the first wave of these changes.

## The 1930 Act

Critics and reformers of the late nineteenth century, as noted earlier, wanted to turn the asylum from a custodial institution into a hospital. They were concerned that the manner in which the asylum was organised prevented this. The practice of certification was deemed particularly problematic. This practice, it was argued, delayed treatment of the insane until a point where they were effectively beyond treatment. This view was based on a very common belief of the time, that only early treatment of mental illness could be successful. What the reformers wanted, then, was a way of speeding up the admission procedures and usually this was felt to require the removal of the need for compulsory certification. Changes in this direction originally began in the private sector. However, legislative changes brought about legal alternatives by the end of the nineteenth century.

The main break came in 1924 when a Royal Commission on Lunacy and Mental Disorder (The Macmillan Commission) was set up. The commission was put together to examine the issue of wrongful detention in public asylums, following a bungled attempt to calm public concern regarding this issue. However, the actual scope of its enquiry and its recommendations spread much wider than this problem. It became a fundamental review of mental health provision. The Commission presented its report in 1926. Its overwhelming message was that psychiatry is a branch of medicine and should be both more integrated with and more akin to the other branches. It argued that the asylum system was too custodial and suggested a shift in the emphasis of psychiatry towards prevention and treatment. Moreover, it criticised the interdependency of the asylums with the Poor Law, on the grounds that such interdependency was not common amongst other branches of medicine. Mental illnesses are the same as physical illnesses, the report argued, and should be thought of, provided for and treated in much the same way. Finally, the need for early treatment and thus circumvention of the certification mechanism was recognised. One would not wait for legal approval to treat another serious illness, it was argued, so why do so with mental illness?

Four specific recommendations were put forward by the commission. First, it was suggested that a system for voluntary admission of patients be added to the system of compulsion. Second, it recommended that provision be made for a proper separation of old (chronic) and new cases. Third, it recommended better after-care facilities. Finally it argued for a shift in the institutional location of provision, from the asylum to the general hospital, and for a dual system of inpatient and outpatient facilities.

Some of this was implemented in the 1930 Mental Treatment Act. This act made public provision for outpatients and aftercare possible, and it introduced three distinct statuses for psychiatric patients: voluntary, temporary and certified. The legal definition of certified patients remained as it was. Temporary patients were compulsorily admitted to hospital for a maximum of six months, without certification. Grounds for admission on this basis were that immediate treatment must be in the best interest of the patient. Voluntary patients were those who applied in writing for their own admission. They had the right to discharge themselves with only seventy-two hours notice. As Figure 3.4 shows, this group grew most rapidly in the period immediately following the act.

Another interesting aspect of the 1930 Mental Treatment Act was that it called for a change in terminology. Following the act, 'asylums' were to be referred to as 'mental hospitals'; 'paupers' were to be referred to as 'rate-aided' persons/patients; and 'lunatics' were to be referred to as 'persons of unsound mind' or 'patients'. This terminological change clearly indicates a

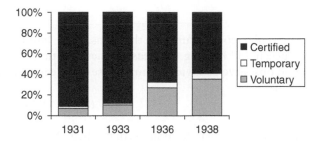

*Figure 3.4* Legal status of admissions to county and borough mental hospitals.
Source: Busfield, J. (1986) *Managing Madness*, London, Unwin Hyman.

conceptual change. There was a concern both to *medicalise* and *humanise* pauper lunatics.

Busfield suggests three key causes for these changes. The first involves the break up of the Poor Law. The policies advocated by the MacMillan commission were strictly opposed to the ideas of the Poor Law and contradicted both its spirit and its operation. If the Poor Law had remained in place then the recommendations of the commission could not have been implemented. But the Poor Law was collapsing by the 1920s and was being replaced by the first developments of what later became the welfare state.

The second factor informing the 1930s reforms was the emergence of what Busfield calls 'office psychiatry'; that is, doctors dealing with milder 'nervous' problems, privately, in consulting rooms outside of asylums. The growth of such practices can be accounted for, in part, she argues, by the dissatisfaction of low-status asylum doctors who wished to improve their situation. The attraction of office psychiatry was that it catered for an exclusively wealthy client base who valued and were prepared to pay for the discretion private practice offered and for the opportunity to avoid the stigma and poor treatment associated with certification and the asylum. The significance of the emergence of office psychiatry was threefold. First, it widened the definition of mental problems to a group of people who required help, but not incarceration. This helped to change public and political perceptions of mental illness, thereby laying the ground for the way of thinking which we see in the 1930 Act. Second, it began to shift the balance of the types of cases dealt with by professional psychiatry in the direction of the neuroses. Again this contributed to the sort of rethinking involved in the 1930 Act. If psychiatry was dealing more with neuroses then its organisation needed to be rethought. Finally, it pointed to ways of working with patients (i.e. psychological methods) which could be organised on an outpatient basis. Asylums, by this point, had become very closely bound up with physical forms of treatment.

A third factor contributing to the changes embodied in the 1930 Act was the experience of shell shock during First World War. The term 'shell shock' was used to refer to a range of symptoms experienced by some soldiers, including:

> ... paralyses and muscular contractures of the arms, legs, hands and feet, loss of sight, speech and hearing, choreas, palsies and tics, mental fugues, catatonia and obsessive behaviour, amnesia, severe sleeplessness, and terrifying nightmares.
>
> (Stone 1986, 251)

The initial reaction of the military was to assume that 'shell shock' was a ploy of malingerers, and the recommendation was that these malingerers be court martialled and then shot. The problem was too big to be treated in this way, however. Too many soldiers were affected. Furthermore, it affected persons of too high a status. Officers from 'good' backgrounds were affected – a medical solution was needed.

Early medical approaches tended to rely upon biological and materialist theories of mind but these proved problematic. One prominent theory, for example, drew upon a notion of inherited mental degeneracy but this could not be applied to the many respectable officers, from influential backgrounds, who were affected. Other theories tended to rely upon a notion that exploding bombs in some way created lesions in the nervous system or brain, but these failed to explain the fact that many of those affected had never been close to exploding bombs or even combat. The door was therefore open to the psychologically inclined, all of whom were to argue, in one way or another, that shell shock symptoms were the effect of the mental trauma of war.

Although not everybody accepted the psychological perspectives many did and, as Stone (1986) notes, this allowed shell shock to be of considerable historical importance. This importance lay in two main directions. In the first instance, shell shock opened the door to ideas about neurosis and psychotherapy, and to the theories of psychoanalysis and psychology. Such ideas had been in circulation before the war but they had not been appropriated to any great extent in Britain, particularly not in the medical profession. Neurosis was a very low status problem for a psychiatrist to have to work with, and psychoanalysis was a low status discipline. The tides turned with shell shock however. Neuroses became important and the inability of biological psychiatry to say or do much in relation to them was the cause of much embarrassment and reprobation. Every respectable psychiatrist needed a psychological (as well as a biological) perspective. Furthermore, the psychologists and psychoanalysts had a golden opportunity to get a foot in the door, both in the sense of carving out a professional space for themselves and by publicising their ideas to a wide and now receptive audience. Neuroses and arguments about their environmental causes had to be taken seriously.

The second major effect of shell shock was that it created a pressure for reform of existing psychiatric services. Up to this point, the main users of psychiatric services were paupers, who enjoyed a low status and attracted little concern. Soldiers were using services now, however, and there was a feeling that they deserved something better. Moreover, there were many of them, more than the asylum system could cope with, and this called for an innovative response. In particular there was a thrust towards the removal of compulsory certification, the introduction of voluntary status patients, and the growth of outpatient facilities. As Stone puts it:

> ... historians of psychiatry have tended to overlook the fact that the boom in out-patient facilities after the First World War began as an attempt to deal with over a 100000 neurasthenic ex-servicemen suffer-ing from the after effects of shell shock – a flood of cases which reached its peak only in 1922. The Ministry of Pensions was forced to set up over 100 treatment centres in an effort to cope with this situation and many of these began to take on civilian day patients soon after the war ended.
>
> (Stone 1986, 246)

The relationship of these pressures and changes to the provisions of the 1930 Act are clear. Indeed Stone has argued that shell shock was the single most important factor behind the changes introduced by the act.

## After the 1930 Act

The period immediately after the 1930 Act was a time of considerable transformation. Busfield (1986) identifies three main directions of change. In the first instance, she argues that the act itself, particularly the provision for voluntary admissions, led to a further change in attitudes and percep-tions concerning mental illness and, consequently, to changes in practice. Many of the most obvious apparatuses of restraint were gradually removed and some effort was made to make mental hospitals more pleasant. This change was doubtless a response to the dissonance between voluntary status and forms of restraint. Related to this, open door policies were intro-duced which allowed at least some patients to walk more freely around the hospital and even in its grounds. By the 1950s, most hospitals had at least some open door wards (ibid.). In addition, connections between the hospi-tal, its surrounding community and the families of inmates began to be forged. This involved both bringing the family and community into the hospital for visits, and allowing inmates out for visits. The strict segregation that had been in place since the middle of the nineteenth century began to give way.

The second axis of transformation involved new therapeutic innovations. From the late 1930s a range of new treatments began to emerge. At first there were the coma and convulsion therapies, such as insulin coma therapy and electro-convulsive therapy (ECT). Later developments included lobotomy and leucotomy. These treatments are all biological in character. They assume that mental illnesses have a biological cause and attempt to cure them by inducing biological changes. And it is fair to say that most significant new developments of this time were biological. The upper hand that shell shock afforded the psychological approaches was relatively short-lived. There were, however, one or two psychological innovations at this time. The most famous of these is the idea of the therapeutic communities, which were developed largely out of the experience of working with shell-shocked soldiers. These communities encouraged patients to take a more active role in their own recovery and attempted to break down some of the organisational hierarchies of the traditional medical setting (Hinshelwood and Manning 1979). The communities organised by Maxwell Jones and Wifred Bion, respectively, were particularly high profile. It is important to flag these developments, as they connect with the account of later chapters in a fairly direct way. It is also important, for the same reason, to flag the development of so called social psychiatry, which focused upon the relationship of the individual psyche to its wider social environment, and also the family studies and therapeutics associated with the Tavistock Clinic (Miller and Rose 1988). Whilst mainstream psychiatry tended to be biologically centred throughout the twentieth century, in the United Kingdom, this has not been to the exclusion of significant social and psychodynamic currents. Indeed the self-image of British psychiatry very much emphasises eclecticism and open-mindedness, and this is not altogether unreasonable. It is important to add, however, that at least some of the social and psychodynamic input in the UK mental health system also comes from outside of the psychiatric profession as such. Part of the eclecticism of UK mental health services is due to its multi-professional base. And this, as noted above, has expanded significantly in the second half of the twentieth century (Busfield 1986, Rose 1985, 1989, Samson 1995).

Third, psychiatric services were included in the newly formed National Health Service (NHS). At first it was not envisaged that psychiatric services would be included within the NHS. The Minister of Health officially stated this in Parliament in 1943. However, this provoked opposition from the professional body of the psychiatric profession, the Royal Medico-Psychological Society, and by the time of the Health Service White Paper of 1944 psychiatric services were included. The arguments for the inclusion, which were appropriated by the politicians, were based on the view that mental illnesses are the same as physical illnesses and should be treated as such.

## Decarceration

However, an even more drastic change was to follow in the second half of the twentieth century. The old mental hospitals were emptied and closed. 'Care in the community' emerged as the new, dominant aspiration. The first indications of this shift emerged in the recommendations of a Royal Commission on Mental Illness and Mental Deficiency (the Percy Commission), which sat between 1954 and 1957, and the subsequent Mental Health Act of 1959, which called for a shift towards a community-based system of provision. This call was also famously reiterated in 1961 by the Minister for Health, Enoch Powell, at a meeting of the National Association for Mental Health (NAMH) (see Chapter 4). He called for their phasing out and predicted that their numbers would be halved by the mid-1970s, a claim he reiterated one year later in his 'New Hospital Plan' (Rogers and Pilgrim 2001).

In effect, the residential population of mental hospitals had peaked in 1954 and already begun to fall. This was not due to a fall in admissions, however, at least not at first. Admission rates continued to rise into the 1980s. It was due to a sharp rise in discharges and a shortening of the average length of stay, resulting, in many cases, in what has been called the 'revolving door syndrome', in which inmates are discharged after a small stay, only to be read-mitted after a short period, then discharged again and so on (Goodwin 1993).

During this period some alternatives to asylum psychiatry began to emerge. There was a notable increase in the role of primary care, as well as a growth of both psychiatric units in general hospitals and smaller, community-based facilities. Bed numbers in the old hospitals also began to fall. In many respects this was a drift, however, and the goal of fully emp-tying and closing the old hospitals was not pursued aggressively until the 1980s, with most hospitals actually closing in the 1990s.

There are many competing explanations for this shift; too many to review meaningfully here (Busfield 1986, Goodwin 1993, Jones 1972, Prior 1993, Rose 1986, Scull 1984). There is no simple explanation. The mental health field was evolving under the force of its own internal dynamics, generating innovations in practice and ideas. The field was also subject to external pressures and dynamics too, however, the principal of these pres-sures being economic. Most commentators reject Scull's (1984) claim that the initial policy shift towards what he calls 'decarceration' was a response to a 'fiscal crisis of the state' and consequent need to reduce public expendi-ture, not least as there no evidence for any such crisis during the 1950s, at the time of the Percy Commission. However, there is evidence to support the notion that considerations of cost were among the reasons that attracted some early advocates of the policy (Busfield 1986, Goodwin 1993, Rogers and Pilgrim 2001), and the idea of moving treatment out of hospitals and into the community dates back to the 1930s, when public expenditure was a critical issue. Moreover, most commentators concede that there was a fiscal crisis of the state in the United Kingdom in the late 1970s, at the point when decarceration effectively kicked in. If not designed, community care policy was at least implemented by a newly elected neo-liberal government whose key priority was to reduce public expenditure in an effort to resolve a fiscal crisis of the state. Money was important, therefore, and, as Scull suggests, community care does seem to have been envisaged as a cost cutting exercise by those who finally implemented it.

## Scare in the community

Simultaneous with the implementation of community care was a major overhaul of the statutory framework. The 1959 legislation was replaced in 1983, with a new mental health act. And psychiatry was then brought further in line with the rest of the NHS, in the 90s, by means of the 1990 NHS and Community Care Act (Rogers and Pilgrim 2001). The former of these acts, the 1983 Mental Health Act, was shaped in some part by one of the key SMOs examined in this study, MIND, and bore clear traces of their discourse. In addition to tidying up the system, the act paid at least some attention to the rights of key players in the system, including 'patients'. If this represented some progress from the patients' point of view, however, community care was generating a pressure for quite different reforms. It was generating panic and a resurgence, if it had ever gone away, of a control focused framing of 'the problem of mental illness'. Most of the problems were relatively invisible, albeit often tragic. They involved an increased level of hardship for those suffering mental health problems, as well as for their families, friends and other informal carers. A small number of high profile incidents which caught the imagination of journalists, however, served to convey the message that mental patients were a danger to the community. These stories generated public fear and outcry in relationship to community care and government were pressured to respond. Even behind the scenes, however, there was an upward trend in the use of coercive measures in psychiatry during the late 1980s and early 1990s (Rogers and Pilgrim 2001, Sainsbury Centre 1998). Shortfalls in policy and resourcing were being compensated by a tightening of control at the local level.

By the end of the 1990s, even the government was calling community care a failure. In his 1998 policy statement, *Modernising Mental Health Services: Safe, Sound and Supportive*, for example, the Health Minister, Frank Dobson, claimed that

> Care in the community has failed. Discharging people from institutions has brought benefits to some. But it has left many vulnerable patients trying to cope on their own. Others have been left to become a danger to themselves and a nuisance to others. Too many confused and sick people have been left wandering the streets and sleeping rough. A small but significant minority have become a danger to the public as well as themselves.
>
> (Dobson 1998)

This turning point is where the period covered in this book effectively comes to an end. As I make final alterations to this chapter, early in 2005, the issue is not resolved, the panic continues and new controversial legislation is under discussion which would tighten control over those with a range of psychiatric diagnoses.

## Markets and consumers

Not all policy twists over the last decade have served to tighten control, however. A general shift within the NHS, associated initially with Thatcherite neo-liberalism but continued by both Tory and Labour governments, served to introduce internal markets into the NHS and to refashion patients as 'consumers' of health services. In effect, the monopoly of services and top-down bureaucratic control of them once effectively enshrined in the NHS was challenged and a system of tendering for and buying in services introduced. This attracted much criticism from left wing commentators, as well as medical staff. Ironically, however, certain commentators within more radical mental health SMOs express a more ambivalent attitude because, as we will see later, the break up of the NHS monopoly generated opportunities for some of the more innovative projects they wished to see and allowed them to effectively pioneer and tender for such schemes. Moreover, they claim that the introduction of a language and philosophy of consumerism, whilst flawed in some respects, has helped to tip the balance of power slightly in their favour, improving their bargaining power within the system. The customer, so the saying goes, knows best, and these particular customers endorse that view.

## Conclusion

The aim of this chapter has been to set the scene for the analysis which follows by describing the historical emergence of psychiatry in the United Kingdom. Much of the chapter has been devoted to a stretch of history which pre-dates the events and developments discussed in later chapters by a quite considerable chunk of time. However, it is important for us to be mindful of this broader historical sweep if we are to make persuasive interpretations of the recent struggles described in subsequent chapters.

In particular, I hope that the longer-term perspective adopted in this chapter has allowed us to see the degree of struggle and contention, as well as the dynamism, that is endemic in the mental health field. We have seen that medics fought for a monopoly over mental health services; that, by the end of the nineteenth century, they had more or less got it; but that this was only temporarily, since there was an influx of new forms of 'psy' profession in the latter half of the twentieth century. We have also seen that many of the early developments in the mental health field were the result of campaigns by a group of bourgeois reformers, the lunacy reformers, whose opposition to the often brutal regimes of the private madhouses was resisted by medics. We have also seen some evidence of protest by 'alleged lunatics' but

I hope that it has been clear that this group, prior to the second half of the twentieth century, played a very minimal role in struggle, not least on account of the difficult social and political situation they were in. Only an extremely small number of very well-to-do 'alleged lunatics', such as John Percival, had their voices of protest heard, and even then their focus was upon the fact that lunacy was 'alleged'. There was no challenge to the category of lunacy itself, only to its wrongful application in this or that case, and there was little attempt, on behalf of alleged lunatics, to defend the rights of the lunatic. This was to change in the twentieth century.

What the chapter has also done, is to paint a picture of the trend of late twentieth century psychiatry, which furnishes a context for our discussion and analysis of its contention. We have seen a psychiatry divided between different theoretical impulses and aspirations; the drive for a biological psychiatry being dominant but also thrown off course by shell shock and the various forms of social and psychotherapeutic psychiatry and the wider experimentation, in the form of therapeutic communities, that it spawned. We have seen a system of provision in the process of major transformation, as the massive asylum system that was constructed in the latter half of the nineteenth century has been dismantled and as the bureaucratic monopoly of the NHS has been both built up and then knocked down, or at least transformed through marketisation and a consumer model. These trends have created difficulties for those with diagnosed mental health problems but they have also created new opportunities and transformed the structural context wherein lives are lived and projects formulated.

Finally, we have seen about-turns and contradictions with respect to the idea of control. At the start of our period of analysis – the 1950s, the government and medics alike, continuing a trend which begun with the 1930 Mental Treatment Act, were keen to refashion the discourse and practice of psychiatry in a way which emphasised care and cure, challenging the pejorative language and custodial practices of the nineteenth century. The aspiration may still have been the same in the 1990s but there was a very strong pressure on government, fuelled by moral panic, to be seen to be doing the business of control; not just for the sake of the wider communities who might fear the prospect of the mentally ill living amongst them but also for the sake of those mentally distressed persons who found living in the community, without strong support, too difficult and whose lives deteriorated. Care in the community had created a scare in the community. These are the wider dynamics we should be mindful of as we trace our history of contention because these are the wider dynamics which have provided the context and occasion of mobilisation and protest.

# 4 Mental hygiene and early protests
## 1930–60

We saw in Chapter 3 that contention surrounding psychiatry is as old as psychiatry itself. This chapter, which focuses upon the evolution of the field of contention between 1930 and 1960, concentrating particularly upon the 1950s, therefore joins a narrative that is already well under way. The chapter focuses upon four SMOs representing the 'mental hygiene' movement and the dynamics generated within the field of contention which persuaded three of them to merge, in 1946, forming the National Association for Mental Health (NAMH). NAMH are better known these days by their campaign name, MIND, which was adopted in 1972, following a successful campaign of the same name in 1971. Notwithstanding the critiques of more radical SMOs, this post-1972 incarnation of the organisation is known for its critical approach to mental health and for civil rights campaigns on behalf of psychiatric patients in the 1970s and 1980s. In addition, as I show later, its internal network and resources have played a very central role in the history of other, more radical SMOs. In these respects, MIND is different now to the way it was, as NAMH, in the 1940s and 1950s. Although, as I will explain, NAMH's perspective has always been progressive in a sense, it was an uncritical apologist for psychiatry in its early years and was keen to defend the latter against criticism, including the criticism of civil rights protestors. I discuss the radicalisation and transformation of NAMH in Chapter 6. Here I am interested in its formation and its early years, all of which I am going to use as a way of bringing the wider field of contention into focus. The field, here as elsewhere, is my primary concern.

In terms of mental health campaigning, the period from the 1930s to the 1960s belongs to a different era to the post-1960s period. A paradigm shift took place within the field of psychiatric contention between the mid-1960s and the mid-1980s, a shift which is at least partly captured in microcosm in NAMH's aforementioned transmutation in MIND. Assumptions were uprooted, losing their taken-for-granted feel, and new ones took their place. Part of what is interesting about the period between 1930 and 1960 is that it allows us to see this shift. It is the 'before' which allows us to see what is significant and new about the 'after'. As with all paradigm shifts, however, this shift consisted as much in a reframing of earlier ideas and practices, as in a rejection and replacement of them. This adds a further level of interest to the period covered in the chapter. It affords us a fresh perspective upon more recent ideas and practices by revealing their embryonic forms. With this in mind I attempt, throughout the chapter, to maintain a balance between a 'continuist' and a 'discontinuist' portrayal. I will endeavour to depict the period between 1930 and 1960 in a manner which will allow us to see, in the context of the book as a whole, how it both anticipated and differed from what was to follow.

The first section of the chapter discusses the discourse which was embodied both by the early NAMH and its ancestral SMOs: the discourse of the mental hygiene movement. The second section of the chapter extends this by showing how this discourse was embodied in the work of these SMOs. The third section of the chapter focuses upon the formation of NAMH and offers an explanation for it, and this is followed, in the fourth section, with a brief discussion of some of NAMH's early activities. The three sections of the chapter which follow focus respectively upon the political involvement and connections of NAMH, its network links and social capital, and its stance in relationship to the growth of considerable criticism of psychiatry in the 1950s. In this latter context, we will see the first stirrings of a civil rights discourse and movement in the field of psychiatric contention. The chapter ends with a brief conclusion which pulls some of the key arguments of the chapter together.

## Mental hygiene: the discursive foundation of the early NAMH

The NAMH was formed in 1946 out of a merger of three inter-war groups, who each embodied the discourse of mental hygiene: The Central Association for Mental Welfare (CAMW), which had formed as *The Central Association for the Care of Mental Defectives* in 1913, changing their name in 1921; *The National Council for Mental Hygiene* (NCMH), which formed in 1922; and *The Child Guidance Council* (CGC), which formed in 1927. In their early years, these groups differed in focus. The CGC was narrowly concerned with child guidance and the establishment and running of child guidance clinics. CAMW worked primarily through local groups to establish a variety of mental health services, particularly for the 'mentally handicapped', and devoted considerable energy to the encouragement and recruitment of volunteers to run these services. NCMH focused upon education and publicity campaigns at the national level, seeking to disseminate expert advice to a general public it deemed very much in need of it. These differences in focus and remit allowed the groups to operate in a relatively complementary way, without too much overlap, competition or mutual interference. Over time, however, the overlap between them became greater. They increasingly shared constituencies, members and even officers, and this 'structural equivalence' (see Chapter 1) and network overlap bred tension. Differences became points of conflict, which had consequences. Dame Evelyn Fox, the founder member of CAMW, for example, resigned her position as (the first) secretary of the CGC following disagreement. She was opposed to both the growing emphasis upon professional training within the CGC and its failure to treat mental deficiency as a part of child guidance work (Thompson 1998). I will return to these tensions, network overlaps and this structural equivalence later. Presently it would be instructive to unpick the discourse of mental hygiene a little, to give us some insight into this movement.

The practices and ideas behind mental hygiene developed simultaneously, albeit in different forms and under different names, in a number of national contexts in response to similar social changes and the problems they posed (Thompson 1995). The term 'mental hygiene' itself dates back to the mid-nineteenth century, however, and is American in origin. In 1893 Isaac Ray, founder of the American Psychiatric Association, defined it in the following terms:

> ...the art of preserving the mind against all incidents and influences calculated to deteriorate its qualities, impair its energies, or derange its movements. The management of the bodily powers in regard to exercise, rest, food, clothing and climate, the laws of breeding, the government of the passions, the sympathy with current emotions and opinions, the discipline of the intellect – all these come within the province of mental hygiene.[1]

Perhaps the two most famous exponents in the US context were Adolph Meyer and Clifford Beers. The work of both of these campaigners resonates with later developments. Meyer, anticipating aspects of anti-psychiatry and Marxist critique (see Chapters 5 and 6), believed that processes of industrialisation and urbanisation were undermining the mental health of Americans. His conception of the mental life of human beings was biologically rooted but he believed that the hurly burly of social life has a strong and often negative impact upon the human organism and its mental health. Beers, pre-figuring the survivor movement (see Chapters 7–9), had been diagnosed mentally ill and incarcerated before writing a powerful critique of asylums and account of his recovery, *A Mind Which Found Itself*. The resonance is only slight, however. Upon his recovery, Beers advanced a 'pull your socks up' attitude towards the mentally ill and proved unsympathetic towards fellow patients, a far cry from the later survivor movement. Moreover, the emphasis upon social aetiology and bio–psycho–social interactions within mental hygiene, though very progressive for its time, was framed rather differently within this discourse to the way in which it would be framed by psychiatric radicals from the 1960s onwards. The dangers of industrialisation and urbanisation were framed primarily in terms of a fear of the impending collapse of civilisation and social order. Mental disorder was perceived to be linked to moral decline, particularly amongst the working class. Moreover, there was a strong concern within the discourse upon efficiency and effectiveness. Mental hygiene literature tended to emphasise loss of working days and the threat to economic and military inefficiency caused by mental health problems and called for mental health promotion as much on these grounds as any other (Rose 1985).

The American sociologist, Kingsley Davis, was a contemporary of the movement. He argued that it embodied and extended both the Protestant work ethic and the reforming zeal rooted in that ethic:

> ...mental hygiene, being a social movement and a source of advice concerning personal conduct, has inevitably taken over the Protestant ethic inherent in our society, not simply as the basis for conscious preachment but also as the unconscious system of premises upon which its 'scientific' analysis and its conception of mental health itself are based.
>
> (Davis 1938, 56)

In other words, whilst the proponents of mental hygiene were advancing what, in good faith, they took to be a scientific definition of mental health and a scientific analysis of the conditions most conducive to its maximisation, they were unwittingly framing this science in terms of a religiously based ethos whose claims were not subject to the rigours of scientific investigation. There was a moral basis to mental hygiene but it was so deeply engrained that the hygienists and their fellow travellers could not see it. They simply took it for granted. Moreover, this ethos was socially specific. It was the ethos of the white, western middle class. The 'civilisation' that the hygienists exalted was Western civilisation, a social order perceived to be superior to both its own barbarous past and the more 'primitive' forms of life of non-western societies. However, the fact of living in a Western society was not sufficient to guarantee a civilised disposition. Mental hygienists were keen to promote 'mental health' and prevent any 'slipping' amongst their own, middle-class ranks. And degeneracy and inefficiency amongst the working class was a major preoccupation. Less respectable elements amongst the working class were deemed to be a threat to civilisation. Their lifestyles were deemed unhealthy and potentially socially damaging. Finally, this discourse embodied relatively stereotyped views of both gender and sexuality. Sexual 'deviation', for which read anything sexual with the exception of genital intercourse between married couples, was identified as a major source of degeneration and social collapse, and thus as a threat.

To illustrate some of these points, we can reflect briefly upon some of the claims of the prominent British hygienist, T.S. Clouston, as outlined in his book of 1906, *The Hygiene of Mind* (on Clouston see Beveridge 1991) A central theme in this book, as more widely in the hygienists' discourse, is the importance of good manners for mental health:

> [the importance of good manners] in Mental Hygiene is twofold – first the influence of the good or bad manners of one child on another, and second, the influence of the constant practice and habit of good

manners on the mind of the child who practices them. Without denying that amongst the educated classes, children come naturally and by hereditary by a certain tendency towards good manners and polite behaviour, yet it is certain that there are such children whose manners do need forming and who, if they habitually see rudeness of manner, will imitate it.

(Clouston 1906, 102)

Manners, as work by both Elias (1982) and Bourdieu (1984) demonstrate, have played a central role in the establishment of collective identity and distinction amongst the bourgeoisie of Western societies. Lacking the 'blood' that defines the aristocracy they have endeavoured to demarcate themselves from the rabble by way of their culture and cultivation (see also Foucault 1984). Clouston's concern with manners embodies this bourgeois preoccupation. He writes from within a context where bourgeois culture has been naturalised and his efforts to equate good manners with mental health further extend this naturalisation. Interestingly, however, he appears also to wrestle with what Bourdieu (1984) identifies as a central problem of cultural politics: the contradiction between the need to universalise one's culture, so as to establish the cultural foundations of legitimate domination, whilst simultaneously preserving the difference that is essential to distinction. Clouston appears to be attempting to square this circle when he claims that the children of the educated classes tend naturally to come by good manners and polite behaviour. The implication is that working class children do not. All children should be good mannered in Clouston's view, but this comes much easier to some (the middle class) than to others (the working class). The middle class, paradoxically, are deemed 'naturally' more 'cultured' (on this paradox see also Bourdieu 1984).

The above cited passage appears to be aimed at an educated and bourgeois readership, warning them of the danger of contagion from others less civilised but also encouraging them to keep their own house in order. Elsewhere Clouston singles out the working class as the key focus for intervention:

... physical degeneracy is taking place, especially amongst the very poor labouring classes, but also [...] a certain mental degeneracy is occurring in some of them. I do not refer to such decided mental changes as occur in insanity and idiocy. [...] What I mean, is a certain narrowing of the mental horizon in the city-bred, a certain helplessness to cope with economic and social difficulties and a certain limitation of the general view of life which are seen in such persons.

(Clouston 1906, 262)

It is not sufficient for the middle class to keep their own house in order. If civilisation is to be saved then initiatives, akin to those of the physical hygiene movement, must be targeted at working-class households.

In common with many other writers in this tradition, Clouston also focused upon problems of juvenile delinquency, a problem he explained by reference to poor childrearing practices. The child guidance clinics, advocated and pioneered by the CGC, are one good example of the type of intervention initiative which emerged out of this discourse. Child guidance clinics were designed to foster both the children and the child rearing practices which would prevent juvenile delinquency, foster good mental health in children and thereby save civilised society from impending ruin.

It is important to reiterate that mental hygienists believed their views to be scientific. Clouston opens *The Hygiene of Mind* with the claim, 'How science can benefit Life is the greatest practical problem of modern civilisation' (Clouston 1906, v). And he reiterates the factual and scientific basis of his claims throughout. For example:

> There is only one natural mode of gratifying sexual nisus and reproductive instinct, and only one truly social arrangement – that of marriage – while there are many unnatural methods. Science, sociology and Christianity are at one in their conclusions and prohibitions. If natural law is not obeyed we have emotional instability, impairment of manliness and of such social virtues as modesty, purity, control of imagination and true chivalry. It will be observed that I am not now pressing any conventional or moral rules or any social or religious dicta, but the laws of body and mind and purely scientific facts.
>
> (Ibid., 245)

The appeal to scientific fact is important. Clouston, like his other hygienist contemporaries, does not want to debate these issues. They may have been discussed within the scientific community but they have emerged now as facts and there is no room for doubt. They should form the basis for guidelines which responsible middle-class families will follow, and for policies and interventions which are imposed upon the labouring classes. Moreover, every effort should be made to convey these facts and the recommendations based upon them to the wider public. Education and the dissemination of 'propaganda' (a term which had not acquired its contemporary pejorative connotation at this point) were central elements in mental hygiene.

In addition to the promotion of good manners, good child-rearing practices etc., this propaganda effort was intended to change public attitudes towards mental illness and reduce stigmatisation of the mentally ill. This resonates with the present. Stigma is still a major concern for campaigners. However, the hygienist concern with stigma was framed differently. In contrast to contemporary campaigners, who criticise stimatisation because it is, in their view, a morally unjustifiable form of social exclusion, the hygienists objected to it on medical grounds. They believed that early intervention was the key to effective treatment of mental illness. The earlier the intervention, the more likely it is to succeed. Stigma, fear and ignorance were deemed problematic, from this point of view, because it was believed that they make people reluctant to admit to mental health problems, thus delaying treatment and reducing its chances of success. Moreover, it was argued that the families of the mentally ill are reluctant to bring their ill member forward for much the same reason.

For all of its conservativism, in its own way and for its time, the discourse of mental hygiene was progressive. The concern with early treatment and stigma represented new 'leading edge' ideas. But more importantly, whilst they sought to establish the validity of the concept of 'mental illness' in collective consciousness, hygienists sought equally to shift the emphasis of mental health services away from an exclusive focus on 'mental illness' and its treatment, making way for a focus upon the promotion of 'mental health'. In the view of the mental hygienists, the insane must be identified and treated very early on, but more importantly still mental illness must be prevented. This is part of the reason for their concern with juvenile delinquency, bad manners etc. These indications of minor transgression were read as first steps towards a more serious derangement, which, if tolerated, would lead to the latter by way of a process of personal unravelling.

The shift called for by the hygienists was quite dramatic, a paradigm shift, and it had financial implications. The promotion of mental health required the development of services and facilities in the community, including child guidance clinics (in which the CGC had a special interest) and the development of psychiatric social work. This was also consistent with government thinking at that time. Moreover, government accepted the hygienist argument regarding early treatment and were keen to promote the attitudinal changes deemed necessary to achieve this. The rationale for the 1930 Mental Treatment Act, discussed in Chapter 3, was very much rooted in these ideas. The problem of stigmatisation is particularly evident in the parliamentary debates leading up to the Act:

> What we want is to change the attitude of the public towards the idea of mental illness. It should be regarded just as physical illness is regarded, and the public should get the idea that it can be treated, with the hope of effecting an improvement.
>
> (*Parliamentary Debates* 1929–30, 1069,
> Dr Vernon Davies speaking)

> Dr Vernon Davies moved to omit the word 'mental' before 'disorder' [in a Parliamentary discussion of the Bill]. He explained that he did so to free the procedure from the stigma popularly attached to mental disorder and to encourage early application for treatment.
>
> (*British Medical Journal* (*BMJ*) 1930, 423)

## The organisational embodiment of mental hygiene in the United Kingdom

As noted earlier, CAMW, NCMH and CGC varied in their activities initially. They specialised in different aspects of the mental hygiene agenda. Interestingly, however, all were concerned to educate the public in the best ways to maintain and maximise mental health. And all were concerned to remove the stigma attached to mental illness. The activities of the NCMH, for example, were described as follows in the *British Medical Journal* (*BMJ*) in 1928:

> ...the National Council for Mental Hygiene has chosen as its special task the building up of enlightened opinion in relation to mental disorder. The council seeks to improve the mental health of the community, and to this end it endeavours to combat the prevailing ignorance and superstition regarding the true nature of mental disorder which so hamper the work of those concerned with the treatment....
>
> (*BMJ* 1928, 183)

In 1929 the *BMJ* described the remit of CAMW in very similar terms: 'Propaganda and education – the former by means of lectures, films and publications, the latter by means of instruction in psychiatry and allied subjects – are amongst the association's chief activities' (*BMJ* 1929, 126).

And the Feversham Committee's (1939) report on the voluntary sector in mental health, which called for a merger of the organisations and constitutes the foundational document of their new existence as NAMH, made a similar observation in relation to the CGC: 'It has endeavoured to educate the public in the need for child guidance clinics, and to assist in their foundation' (Feversham Committee 1939, 5).

This overlap, which, as noted earlier, became more comprehensive and extensive in the course of the 1930s, was one of the reasons why the three organisations merged into NAMH in the mid-1940s. I will discuss the merger shortly. First, however, it is important to note that NAMH very much continued the hygienist emphasis in their early years. The Feversham Report, which was effectively the blueprint for the new organisation, defined their remit in the following way, for example:

1   To educate the public in an understanding of mental health, and to promote and organise cooperation of all activities in this sphere.
2   To work for and promote the preservation of mental health and the prevention and treatment of mental disorders and defects amongst both adults and children.
3   To work for and promote the study of and research into mental health, mental disorders and defects, and to obtain and make records of and disseminate information.

4   To promote the training of workers in the mental health field and
the establishment of standard qualifications.

(Feversham Committee 1939, 232)

Moreover, the problematisation of lifestyle, particularly working class
lifestyles, remained a persistent theme, as the following quotation from an
editorial of *Mental Health*, the journal of the newly formed NAMH,
illustrates:

> ...the plight of the routine manual worker whose leisure is never spend
> in any creative occupation. This is nowadays easy to understand: mass
> production in work does not encourage initiative, and the offer of a
> holiday or leisure where details are arranged for him attracts the indi-
> vidual whose initiative has thus been sapped. Hence the growth of
> 'mass produced' or spoon-fed leisure – listening to music rather than
> playing, watching games rather than taking part – and the growth of
> sensational reading or film going. Other civilisations than ours have,
> of course, had their bread and circuses in their decline. The ability to
> amuse oneself alone, with hands or brain, is getting rarer.
>
> Yet the would-be reformer is faced with a paradox – if he encourages
> means of using leisure constructively, he may help in spoon-feeding and
> leaving no room for initiative. What is he to do? He must be satisfied
> with creating opportunities for leisure to be spent and hoping that the
> opportunities will gradually and occasionally be taken. It will be slow.
>
> (*Mental Health* 1950, 1–2)

In the following decade radicals such as Herbert Marcuse and the anti-
psychiatrist, R.D. Laing, would be making very similar claims, albeit
embellished by reference to Marx, Hegel and others, under the rubric of
'alienation' (see Chapter 5). Workers are no longer just alienated in work,
Marcuse (1986) argued. Mass culture alienates them in their leisure also.
Where Marcuse and Laing were engaging in a critique of society, however,
NAMH were problematising the workers affected by this process. They
aimed to encourage workers to take up constructive leisure pursuits which
would keep their minds active and therefore healthy.

The reference to film in the above passage indicates a new angle that
mental hygiene was acquiring, moreover. Very soon after their formation
NAMH recognised that, '...cinema is becoming one of the most important
influences in the modern world' (*Mental Health* 1967, 7(2), 47). This could
be an influence for the better, they believed, but it could equally be to the
detriment of the mental health of the population. Partly this was because
cinema was perceived as a passive activity. Audiences consumed it in a
pre-packaged form, rather than being actively involved in its production –
Marcuse might have said that it was 'alienating' on just these grounds. In
addition, there was a concern that both children and the mentally ill are

adversely affected by film, lacking critical faculties and being incapable of fully distinguishing between fantasy and reality. On top of this, however, there was a concern that cinematic interest in psychology, psychiatry and related issues results in misrepresentation of them and thereby misleads the public. Considering the hygienist belief that ignorance and misinformation regarding psychiatry and mentally illness are causes of delayed treatment, which in turn is a cause of potentially curable problems becoming incurable, this was deemed a major problem. For this reason a 'Film Visiting Committee' was formed in 1947, whose purpose was to: '...give valuable technical guidance and help in relation to producing, and also in avoiding inaccurate presentations which would tend to vulgarise psychology and give the public a false idea of its possibilities' (*Mental Health* 1967, 7(2), 47).

In 1948, the Film Visiting Committee joined forces with members of the *British Film Academy*, giving rise, in 1963, to the *Mental Health Film Council*. Their reviews were generally published in *Mental Health*. The following review for 'The Upturned Glass', reproduced in full here, gives a flavour of the nature of the early reviews:

> In this film once again psychology only appears in conjunction with the abnormal and the criminal. It is an exciting film and much of the photography is exceedingly clever, but it would be difficult to leave the cinema without the feeling, conscious or not, that an understanding of man's mental processes is akin to a knowledge of the occult and brings in its sinister train wickedness, violence and murder.
>
> A brain surgeon plots deliberately and brutally to kill a woman in a horrible situation; this same man, who is also a lecturer in criminal psychology, deludes himself into believing that he is a dispenser of justice on a divine scale; and the casting of James Mason as the criminologist ensures that this character shall be subtly played in all its unpleasantness. Psychological vocabulary is used throughout the film and much is made of the technical term 'paranoid'. The surgeon is called 'paranoid' frequently, apparently because of his conviction that he is called on to dispense justice, and it is stated as a psychological fact that a paranoid always feels compelled to tell someone of his crime. 'Obsessional' too is another favourite term in the film, used more or less as a synonym of 'paranoid'.
>
> Dilys Powell in the *Sunday Times* has called *The Upturned Glass* 'a neat, empty story of murder with the modish psychological trimmings', but they are very large trimmings indeed and, for the most part, false and frightening. PW.
>
> (*Mental Health* VII(3), 83)

The review is interesting because it allows us to see how the work of framing within the discourse of mental hygiene taps into tacit assumptions akin to Davis's (1938) aforementioned unconscious ethos. The sense of the review rests upon a taken-for-granted distinction between lay and professional understandings of psychology and an assumed duty of the expert to protect the lay public from themselves. Lines such as '...it is stated as psychological fact...' and '"Obsessional" too...', for example, are clearly identifying errors. The reader is supposed to understand that it is '[wrongly] stated as psychological fact' and that the term 'obsessional' is [mis]used more or less...'. But this is not stated. The sentences embodying these claims make little sense unless one reads them in these ways but more importantly the writer draws upon a tacit 'typification' (Schutz 1967) of film makers/audiences as uninformed and of hygienist critics as experts, not doubting that the full meaning of his or her claims is clear. This also has the effect of positioning the reader as an expert, qualified to judge the errors of the layman, and the review presupposes its reader's willingness to take up this position for its meaning and effect. If they are not bothered about misuse of psychological terminology then the exasperated tone of the review will fall flat, as it would if the reader feels unqualified to have an opinion on such matters. The review invites and requires collusion for its full meaning and effect. Furthermore, prefacing remarks such as '...once again...' indicate that this is one more example of a worrying trend. The review positions itself as a 'chapter' in an ongoing and worrying narrative which the reader is assumed to be following. What is particularly worrying about the film is that it is not an isolated case. Finally, note that the review is constructed within certain 'structures of relevance' (ibid.) such that it only serves the purposes of and only makes sense to those with an interest in guiding the common woman/man. It is not, to offer a contrast, structured to suit the needs of the prospective cinemagoer or film connoisseur. These readers would need different information about the film and would want their attention directing to other aspects of it. They would not be interested in that fact that '...psychological vocabulary is [mis]used...' or that '...much is [incorrectly] made of [our scientific and] technical term...' because these are aesthetically irrelevant observations. From the perspective of cinematic aesthetics the review completely misses the point and misunderstands the nature of cinematic texts, whose value is not ordinarily judged in terms of scientific accuracy. There is no appreciation of 'artistic licence'. However, the *Mental Health Film Council* were not framing their reviews from an aesthetic point of view. They were framing them from a hygienist point of view, drawing upon the assumptions, 'typifications', 'relevances' and imperatives of the hygienist discourse.

NAMH were not only interested in criticising films; they were also interested in making them. Some educative films on mental health, shown at mental health exhibitions and during 'mental health weeks', had been made by NAMH's ancestral groups and the early NAMH continued to show these films at their conferences and events. With the formation of the *Mental Health Film Council*, however, the involvement with film intensified. The Council became interested in the technical process of film making and, recognising the lack of practical expertise amongst its membership, began to organise courses and events on film making. This generated a glut of new hygiene films, some of which made their way into mainstream picture houses as a 'warm up' to the feature film.

These observations on cinema have an interesting and important bearing for our understanding of campaigning. They illustrate the different forms of competence and resources presupposed by different arenas of struggle. In order to launch a successful campaign in the cinematic field, NAMH needed to forge links with relevant agents (e.g. the British Film Academy) and acquire the requisite forms of competence for effective action in the cinematic field. It was able to this because it was rich in transferable resources but that does not alter the fact that resources and connections had to be mobilised and converted, and new skills acquired.

## The formation of NAMH

The merging of CAMW, NCMH and CGC into NAMH followed a recommendation in the (1939) report of the Feversham Committee: *The Voluntary Mental Health Services*. The committee had a broad membership which included members of all three groups and a fourth, *The Mental Aftercare Association for Poor Persons Convalescent or Recovered from Institutions for the Insane* (formed in 1879 as *The Aftercare Association for Poor and Friendless Female Convalescents on Leaving Asylums for the Insane*), who were also recommended to partake in the merger. The *Mental Aftercare Association*, who remain active today under the abbreviated name, *MACA*, resisted the merger because they believed that a merged organisation would be too big and bureaucratic to care properly for the needs of individuals, and also because they wanted both to maintain their independence and to avoid closer cooperation with the state. However, the other three agreed to merge.

The Feversham Report was effectively a blueprint for the new, merged organisation. It suggested a name for the new group (*The National Council for Mental Health*), which was adopted in a slightly altered form (*The National Association for Mental Health*). It suggested a date for amalgamation, which was delayed until 1946 by the Second World War, although the groups did work together between 1942 and 1946 as *The Provisional Council for Mental Health*. And it suggested both a constitution for the organisation and the set of aims (cited earlier). In addition, Earl Feversham himself took up the chair of the new organisation from its inception until his death in 1963.

On the basis of the report and related documentation, I suggest that the processes leading up to, necessitating and bringing about the merger can be understood at five interacting levels, each of which is a dimension of the field of psychiatric contention. In the first instance, we must consider factors relating to the internal development of the groups themselves.

CAMW are particularly significant in this respect. They started out as a philanthropic, voluntary organisation for working with 'mental defectives'. Over time, however, their focus began to shift away from 'mental deficiency' towards the more fashionable concerns of mental hygiene. This put them in an uncomfortably competitive position with NCMH. Moreover, an emphasis upon the professionalisation of care within the group, in the form of psychiatric social work, meant that it was beginning to outgrow its role and place in the voluntary sector and needed to find either a new role, a new space in which to play its existing role or both (Thompson 1995). This was a problem which all of the groups experienced to some extent. Each was outgrowing its original remit and needed to take stock of who and what it was and what it hoped to achieve.

The second level that we need to consider is that of the interaction between the groups. As I have already suggested, changes within the individual groups, which caused them to converge in terms of ideas, practices and aims, led to increased overlap and competition between them. This created tension between the groups and greatly reduced their efficiency. Some practices were unnecessarily duplicated, whilst others, which could have been provided given the available resources, were not because resources were tied up in duplicated practices. This state of affairs was noted in 1930 by the Commonwealth Fund but the chance of amalgamation or closer cooperation at this stage was thwarted by the (aforementioned) antagonism between CAMW and CGC. The issue emerged again, however, in a strong criticism of the poor organisation of social work in a report by Political and Economic Planning (PEP 1937a,b, 1939). The Feversham Committee was set up partly as a result of this report and a key theme of its own report was the waste and lack of efficiency created by competition and lack of coordination between the groups. Some solution to this problem had to be found, the report argued, and merger was the solution opted for.

These first two levels clearly interact with one another. Inter-group dynamics impact upon each of the groups involved, prompting them to make changes in their individual structure. And changes in each of the individual groups, whether prompted by inter-group dynamics or by something else, impact upon inter-group dynamics, since changes in one party to an interaction have implications for the other parties. Specifically, convergence in aims and activities lead to greater structural equivalence as the groups forged an increasingly similar profile of interdependencies. And this generated both competition and network overlap – of constituencies, membership and even personnel – between the groups, which, in turn, generated conflict and inefficiency. It was more difficult for the groups to 'agree to disagree' when their common ties of dependency meant that success for one (e.g. in securing funds) was failure for the others. The dynamics of this interaction could have propelled the field in any of a number of directions but, as noted earlier, whilst conflict between the groups prevented merger at an earlier point of time, the inefficiency it created was effectively recognised, a mechanism of arbitration effected (the Feversham Committee) and this motivated a merger between three of the four main players in the field at this time. NAMH, in this respect, was very much a product of the dynamics of the field of psychiatric contention in the 1930s.

We can deepen this account by reference to the value-added model discussed in Chapter 2. The problems generated by conflict between the groups can be theorised as a 'strain' which, having been 'framed' as a problem which could be resolved though merger, motivated three of the groups to join forces. As the value-added model predicts, however, strain and framing in themselves were insufficient to prompt the merger. Animosity between the groups prevented merger at an earlier time, and the Second World War delayed the merger when it had finally been agreed upon. In the latter case, we might say that war generated an environment which was not 'structurally conducive' to merger, whilst the early animosity, read as a lack of solidaristic network links between the groups, was a problem at the level of mobilisation structures. The PEP reports which prompted the formation of the Feversham Committee list any number of 'precipitating factors' and are themselves precipitating factors insofar as they articulate strains and call for a resolution. Finally, the involvement of both PEP and the Feversham Committee are both examples of significant third party responses. Had any of these factors been different, NAMH may not have been formed, at least not in the way that it was.

The field of psychiatric contention did not exist in a vacuum, however. It was located within a wider mental health field, which was, in turn located in a broader welfare field, which was in turn located in a national societal field. Each of these levels were interacting too, having a mutual impact upon one another. And this too was important in terms of the merger and formation of NAMH. The changes that the groups were undergoing and the need for their coordination were greatly influenced, for example, by the early development of the Welfare State, which was undermining the role of voluntary groups by instituting professional, public sector welfare agencies. The groups were forced to change because the wider environment in which they were interacting was changing. The formation of the Welfare State generated a strain for traditional voluntary groups by effectively displacing them. We see this clearly in Feversham's report. Much of the discussion in the report focuses upon the appropriate place of voluntary groups in what was identified at the time as the new, welfare era. Furthermore, these institutional changes were giving rise to cultural and discursive changes. As one of the key early activists in NAMH, Edith Morgan, notes: 'Old-style charity was seen as demeaning and redundant in the new welfare state. Mind[2] had to put a convincing case for a new role for voluntary organisations' (Morgan 1997).

These transformations in the welfare field, in turn, were part of the general shift within capitalist society, motivated at the governmental level by the perceived threat of class-based political conflict (Busfield 1986, Gough 1979, Scull 1984). The interventionist state, with its minimal and punitive system of poor law provision, was giving way to a welfare state under the pressure created by a growing labour movement and corresponding threat of social unrest (Busfield 1986, Gough 1979).

We should not read this chain of interaction in a purely top-down way, however. The activities of voluntary associations, such as the hygienist groups, provided an infrastructure and model that the welfare state was built upon and drew from. Moreover, some of the hygienists had been campaigning for the professionalisation of the services they provided (opposed by others) and offered the training necessary for professionalisation (Thompson 1995). They were amongst the voices calling for what became the welfare state and thus they had some role in bringing about the changes in the welfare field which, in turn, generated change in both their own field of contention and their individual organisations. They were victims of their own success, although of course their own campaigning influence was only one amongst a number of factors generating pressure for these wider changes and there is no reason to believe that it was decisive.

The concept of 'interaction' is crucial to my account here. It is intended to capture the sense in which groups were active agents who pursued projects and responded to wider events in a purposive fashion, whilst indicating that they were part of a wider environment of agents whose activities impacted upon them and which they were forced to respond to, in the respect that carrying on as usual was not an option. The environment is a constraint here but I have argued that it too 'interacts' with the groups in the respect that they play a part, however small, in changing it. Moreover, claiming that groups change in response to events in their wider environment is only a way of affirming their purposive agency. We would question the agency of a group or individual who continued to act in an identical manner when everything around them was changing. It is of the essence of agency to be able to respond meaningfully to events in one's environment.

## Interventions in the mental health field

The early NAMH, as described by a female psychologist who joined in the late 1950s, was staffed by middle-class ladies 'of a certain age', who conducted their affairs in a polite but formal manner:

> The NAMH was very much a women's organisation in those days. The only man on the staff was a psychologist who was rarely seen at headquarters. [...] It was a revelation to come down to tea, served with some formality by the 'tea lady', and join a circle of ladies wearing an assortment of footwear, the like of which I had seen only in my grandmother's photographs – and this in the era of winklepickers and stiletto heels!
>
> (Husain 1992)

The genteel atmosphere did not impede the organisation from pursuing its hygienist agenda with vigour and success, however. This involved much work within the mental health field itself. NAMH took over the services of its ancestral groups and continued to develop new ones. In 1946, it was running 11 agricultural hostels for 'mentally handicapped' men, 2 homes for 'mentally defective' children, 2 holiday homes for 'mental defectives' and inmates of mental hospitals as well as a convalescent home for 'epileptics' (MIND 2004). In 1947 a further convalescent home, an approved school, a home for old people and a home for 'pre-delinquent children' were added to this list (ibid.). In addition, NAMH offered courses on mental health to a range of professional groups (many NAMH members were drawn from the ranks of these groups), including: doctors responsible for diagnosing 'mental deficiency', teachers of 'educationally subnormal' children, psychologists, health workers, social workers, psychiatric social workers and educational psychologists (ibid.). They organised mental health exhibitions which explained, advocated and advertised their models of good psychiatric services to a range of interested and relevant parties. Moreover, they promoted communication, information sharing and debate amongst professionals and interested volunteers. This involved the publication of a wide range of books on mental health issues and the amalgamation of CAMW's journal, *Mental Welfare* – previously *Studies in Mental Inefficiency* – with NCMH's journal, *Mental Hygiene*, to create a new journal, *Mental Health*. Finally, they held annual conferences in London, which were regularly addressed and attended by politicians, as well as professionals and volunteers. The conferences enjoyed a good reputation in the wider mental health field and were always very well attended. Indeed, attendance figures regularly exceeded 2000 (Jones 1972, 321).

The importance of the conference, which I will return to at a number of points in this book, is indicated by the fact that, in 1961, the Minister for Health, Enoch Powell, selected it as the first platform for announcing plans to speed up the shift to deinstitutionalised care called for by the *1959 Mental Health Act* (see Chapter 3 and below) by implementing a massive reduction in mental hospital beds and beginning a closure programme for the country's mental hospitals. It was traditional for health ministers to make the inaugural speech at the NAMH conference during this period and it was usual for them to take the opportunity to 'sound out' new ideas (ibid.). The contents of the 1961 address were so radical, however, that the speech and its implications remained a talking point in the pages of *Mental Health* throughout the 1960s.

NAMH's efforts were not restricted to the mental health field, however. I have already discussed their cinematic ventures. And as the earlier reference to the Powell speech indicates, they formed connections with and were active within the parliamentary field too. This point needs to be fleshed out.

## Interventions in the parliamentary field

The parliamentary field was and still is important in relation to the mental health field because much of what occurs in the latter is framed by laws and policies formulated in the former. A consequence of this situation is that psychiatric skills and credentials are not sufficient for agents to achieve a transformation of psychiatry. Would-be reformers must have the competence and resources appropriate for parliamentary intervention. NAMH were both plugged in and tuned in, in this respect. I have already noted the involvement of government ministers in their annual conferences for example. By means of this channel they enjoyed direct contact with government. Government sought advice from NAMH and used the conference as a way of consulting with interested parties, whilst NAMH members were afforded the privilege of hearing about new policy developments in their early stages, from the horse's mouth, with an opportunity to respond and ask questions. In addition to this, however, they were chaired by a succession of Lords. Their first chair, as noted earlier, was the Earl of Feversham, who was followed successively by Lord Balniel (1963), Christopher Mayhew MP (1969), Lady Bingley (1978) and Lord Ennals (1984), before the post passed outside of the circle of immediate political influence. Moreover, their president from 1946 to 1990 was the Rt Hon R.A. Butler MP, who was succeeded by Lord Ennals (1990), followed by Lord Bragg (2000). The list of notables could be extended but what is more important is the fact that at least some of these notables mobilised their connections and status to advance the NAMH cause. Through Feversham's seat in the Lords, for example, NAMH enjoyed direct access to and participation in the second chamber. A brief summary of his main political achievements, which gives some clue as to the way in which he was able to use his political advantage, was provided in his (1963) obituary in *Mental Health*:

> In 1958 he initiated the first debate in the House of Lords on the Royal Commission's Report on the Law Relating to Mental Illness and Mental Deficiency. He attended all the sittings when the Mental Health Act of 1959 was before the Lords, speaking on a number of amendments. In February 1960 it was at his instigation that the Younghusband Report was first debated. Last year, in July he initiated a debate on the working of the Mental Health Act.
>
> (Appleby 1963)

These parliamentary links were consolidated at two further levels. First, the mental hygiene issues raised by NAMH and their efforts to educate the public were in line with government thinking of that time. They enjoyed a discursive affinity. If we examine the Parliamentary debates leading up to the 1959 *Mental Health Act*, for example, it is clear that there was a cross-party agreement that the public needed educating with respect to mental health and illness. The hygienist discourse which had informed the earlier, 1930 *Mental Treatment Act* was, undoubtedly, part of the reason for this. However, the shift towards community-based settings that the 1959 act recommended created an additional pressure, Greater public tolerance towards mental illness was required if the policy was going to work:

> The idea of caring for the mentally disordered in the community is still often accepted only as a principle. Too often it becomes a different matter if a hostel is to be provided in the house next door or even the same neighbourhood.
>
> I think that personal sympathy and help are still too often lacking when compared with the feeling of charity and understanding which are aroused by those who suffer from a physical disability. It is for those who can guide public opinion to show full support for the new attitude which will be required if the plans of the hospitals and local authorities are to succeed.
>
> (*Parliamentary Debates* 1958–59, 919,
> Walker-Smith speaking)

Furthermore, it is clear from the debates that action, in the form of education and propaganda, was believed necessary.

> I would like to know something more about the intentions of the government to embark upon an imaginative campaign to educate the general public more fully than has been the case in the past.
>
> (Ibid., 830, Blenkinsop speaking)

> The Minister has mentioned remedial propaganda. I agree with him. The things said in this House today could be taken to the families of those who have disturbed minds. They could be made known through television, radio and newspapers which cared to approach this matter in a very serious fashion.
>
> (Ibid., 133, Summerskill speaking)

NAMH embraced this task, accepting its necessity on the grounds of both mental hygiene and the demands for public tolerance which a shift to community-based care would create:

> The task of changing public attitudes towards mental disorder is one which the National Association for Mental Health has undertaken because the 1959 Mental Health Act will certainly prove ineffective unless the man in the street understands its implications and is ready to co-operate.
>
> (*Mental Health* 1967, 16(3), 12–13)

Second, there was a financial bond between the NAMH and government. Although they generated money through charity events, NAMH were partially dependent upon central government.

These connections were not incidental to NAMH's structure. Lord Feversham had, after all, been the 'independent' adviser who had recommended the formation of NAMH in the first place. In this respect, the organisation was a political creation whose status as a voluntary rather than a statutory organisation was blurred to say the least – especially if we also consider the political funding it received. And this blurring was carried over from NAMH's ancestral organisations. CAMW, in particular, occupied an ambiguous position (Thomson 1995). In addition to receiving funds from central government, their constitution effectively ensured that half of their executive committee comprised central and local government representatives (ibid.). And their local associations tended to follow suit, co-opting local government representatives to their committees (ibid.). In this respect NAMH was very much formed within a web of interested political parties.

Connections can be both a blessing and a curse. They constitute what Elias (1979) calls a 'balance' of power. Each party can use the other's dependence upon it to influence it. In NAMH's case, the services they provided for government gave them leverage for both putting their views across, being 'in the loop', and securing income. Their dependence upon government gave the latter considerable leverage in relation to them, however, and very much tipped the balance of power. There was a price to be paid for favour. NAMH's decision to take responsibility for the public education proposed by a shift to community care as well as its active defence of psychiatrists and government against criticism should both be read in this light.

## Networks

Political connections were only one aspect of the 'social capital' of the early NAMH, however. They were extremely well-connected within the mental health field itself. In part this was by way of their conferences, journal, services and educational and publicity events, which reached out to and drew in individuals from a range of mental-health-related professions. At a more official level, however, they had a 'medical director' drawn from amongst the upper echelons of the psychiatric profession and their journal was edited by a leading psychiatrist. Furthermore, the members of their ruling council were all drawn either from amongst mental health professionals or, more importantly, from professionals representing a range of other influential organisations including: the *Institute for the Scientific Treatment of Delinquency*, the *Magistrates Association* and three Royal Colleges (Nursing, Physicians and Surgeons).[3] NAMH was 'plugged in' where it mattered.

In addition, a point which will be of more significance later in my account, NAMH was itself a network and generator of networks. Different parties with an interest in mental health became linked through their common involvement in NAMH. It was a network 'bridge', occupying a 'structural hole' (Burt 1992) in the wider national network comprising the mental health field. And this lent it power, importance and influence. Other parties connected to one another through its mediation and depended upon it for this mediation.

The conference, as noted earlier, was very important in this respect. Regularly attended by members of different mental health related professions, as well as volunteers, and regularly addressed by a government ministers, it was a central hub of the mental health field; a place where ideas and practices could diffuse, jumping between professional circles. It was a place where connections between like-minded individuals could be forged, giving rise to new developments and groups. If the mental health field, with all of its internal heterogeneity, nevertheless connected up, then the NAMH conference (along with the *Mental Health* journal) was one reason why it did.

In addition, NAMH bridged local, national and international levels of organisation and interaction, again serving as a conduit for the movement of ideas, practices and resources within and between these levels. At the international level, for example, continuing the links and activities of their ancestral organisations, they organised and hosted, in 1948, the Third Congress of the *International Committee on Mental Hygiene* (*Mental Health* 1947, VI(2), 97 and 1947, VI(3), 65–6) and during that congress helped to set up the *World Federation for Mental Health* – whose annual conferences they subsequently both attended and discussed in *Mental Health*. Moreover, in 1951, along with a number of senior politicians, they attended the first post-war meeting of the *European Committee for Mental Hygiene*, in Switzerland, where they helped to form the *European League For Mental Hygiene* (*Mental Health* 1951, XI(1), 24–6). The function of the international and European associations was to discuss the international dimension of mental health. For example the coordination of international services and national differences in rates of cure, relapse and incidence. But they also served as a bridge, linking national organisations and governments to key international political organisations, such as the *United Nations Educational, Scientific and Cultural Organisation* (UNESCO) and the *World Health Organisation* (WHO). They could, they claimed, both advise and persuade such organisations on matters relating to mental health, much as NAMH were doing at the national level.

Regional offices and local associations were a new development (although CAMW had tended to work locally and Child Guidance Clinics were locally rooted). Both took off in the 1970s (see Figure 4.1) and as such fall outside of the era being examined in this chapter (see Chapter 6). However, it is necessary to at least flag up their significance here. As NAMH

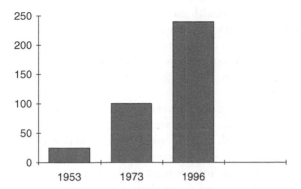

*Figure 4.1* Number of NAMH local associations 1953–96.

Source: The figures for this graph are taken from *Mental Health* 1953, XII(2), *Open Mind* 50, 1991 and personal communication with South Yorkshire MIND regional office.

developed more regional offices and local associations it effectively extended its tentacles geographically, making contact with players in the mental health game whom it would not previously had been connected with and considerably boosting its active membership – since local activism is less costly for activists living at a distance from the geographical centre of the national organisation and local recruitment campaigns can be both more targeted and more effective in terms of securing practical involvement. The extension of its tentacles afforded NAMH an opportunity to spread its message (still essentially a hygienist message until the 1970s) and to cultivate 'good' (i.e. 'mentally hygienic') practices much further than it had previously been capable of. An example of this is a campaign run jointly with the Red Cross in Northamptonshire, between April and October 1963 (*NAMH News* April 1965). Throughout the period, three identified target groups were approached in different ways. First, all local voluntary societies, which held regular meetings, were offered a NAMH speaker to address their group. Second, a number of key groups, known to be respected by the public (including the clergy, the police and teachers), were offered one or half day conferences on mental health issues. As opinion leaders, these groups were felt to be important targets. Finally, the general public themselves were targeted by way of the local media, by open days at the local mental hospital and by campaigners stopping people and distributing leaflets in the street. The campaign finished with an intensive week which included Mental Health Sunday (when information on mental health was spread at church services), a mental health exhibition, film evenings and a one-day conference. The organisers of the campaign used survey methods (before and after) in an attempt to gauge their success. They claimed that the campaign had been successful, although some problems had emerged and the attitudes of the public had proved difficult to determine.

The local associations were essentially autonomous, however, such that, as hubs for diverse local mental health campaigners and other interested parties, they could and sometimes did develop their own agenda. Local associations were and are affiliated to the national body, share its name and abide by a common constitution, but each is a separately registered charity and an independent organisation which determines its own goals and pursues them in its own way.

The links of the local and regional levels to the national level also link those local and regional levels to one another, via the national 'hub', making the national mental health field a 'small world' and potentiating communication and contact between interested parties from remote localities who might not otherwise come into contact with each other. NAMH's local and regional tentacles facilitated more than a mere downward flow of ideas and practices from the (national) centre. They facilitated a flow between localities and secondary networking between these localities. Through its regional offices and more particularly its local associations, NAMH drew even more people into the world of mental health campaigning, and through its own internal network structure, it linked them together – the conference, again, was central in this respect. Moreover, the presence of international links meant that this process was not bound to the national level. Ideas, practices and connections could flow from the local through to the international level and back again. Given the relative autonomy of the local associations this could clearly give rise to more than NAMH were bargaining for.

## Rising contention

I have suggested that NAMH and its ancestral groups, embodying as they did the discourse of mental hygiene, were progressive in many respects, for their time. They sought to change the mental health field, refocusing it such that it was as much about mental health as mental illness, introducing new professions (psychiatric social work and psychology) into it and dragging it away, in both image and reality, from the old asylum system, with its punitive, poor law associations. These progressive ideas were not especially at odds with the ideas of either the psychiatric profession or the government. Indeed both were agreed upon these aims and were happy to work with NAMH in an effort to bring them about. The mental health field was not without its contentious issues at this time, however, nor without more contentious critics. And the reaction of NAMH to these critics is interesting as it draws out more clearly the conservativism within their otherwise progressive stance. In this final section of the chapter, I want to briefly reflect upon these criticisms and NAMH's response.

High profile criticism of psychiatry in the 1950s focused upon two key issues. First, there was a concern about wrongful detention in mental hospitals and the mistreatment of patients therein. There was a strong belief in some quarters that certification was being used to detain groups who were neither mentally ill nor dangerous (danger was commonly associated with certification in the popular conception) including 'spastics', 'the deaf', the old and unmarried mothers. Many of this was brought to public attention by the activities of the National Council for Civil Liberties (NCCL), who had formed in 1934 and targeted certification in one of their first major campaigns. They took several big cases to court, successfully winning the release of their clients and, at the same time, generating a great deal of public concern about certification. This was consolidated, in 1951, when they published a pamphlet, *55000 Outside the Law*, which claimed knowledge of 200 cases of wrongful confinement. Moreover, when, in 1954, a parliamentary committee (the Percy Committee) was formed to look into the possibility of reform of mental health services, a possibility which was actuated in the form of the 1959 Mental Health Act, NCCL, who were asked to give evidence to the committee, were extremely critical. Of all voices at the time, NCCL were perhaps the loudest of those calling for legal reform.

In addition, in 1957, two politicians (one Tory, one Labour), worked together to edit and publish a book, *The Plea for the Silent*, containing eight stories by individuals who had previously been locked in mental hospitals, all alleging wrongful confinement and mistreatment, which had first appeared as letters in their parliamentary mailbags (McI Johnson and Dodds 1957). Each story was critical of the treatment received by the patient and, as the editors themselves pointed out, they were very similar in their details, despite the fact that the individual authors had never met, were from different parts of the country and had been certified by different doctors in different asylums. The book generated a great deal of attention in the press and added considerable weight to the other stories which were emerging at the time.

The stories and testimonies in *The Plea for the Silent* were a far cry from those of contemporary 'survivors' (Crossley and Crossley 2001). And the critique in *55000 Outside the Law* was very different from those which were to follow in the 1960s. The editors of *The Plea*, for example, felt the need to vouch for the probable veracity of their contributors' accounts, anticipating the fact that readers would dismiss the stories of mental patients as delusions. And some reviewers did more or less dismiss the book's critique on these grounds (ibid.). Moreover, there was no sign of the discourse of survivors that we see in contemporary accounts, with its distinctive vocabulary, theories and 'counter-memory' of psychiatric history (ibid. and Chapter 7). The accounts in the book are generally very particularistic, tying their complaints to particular institutions and staff members. In addition, they are and recognise that they are relatively unique. It was extremely rare for patients to express criticism of psychiatry on a public platform at this time, as it had been throughout the history of psychiatry and would be for the next twenty years. Nevertheless, there they were, alongside the NCCL and *55000 Outside the Law*.

In addition to certification and mistreatment, overcrowding in asylums and concerns about their upkeep were also prominent critical themes in public discourse on psychiatry at this time. Labour MP Kenneth Robinson first put this latter issue on the agenda in February 1954 in a Private Members Bill (*Parliamentary Debates* 1953–54). He acknowledged the problems of the legal framework within which psychiatry was enmeshed and noted that it was over a quarter of a century since Parliament had debated matters relating to mental health, despite the enormous changes that the practice of psychiatry had been undergoing. His main concerns, however, were the 'serious overcrowding of mental hospitals', the 'high proportion of obsolete and unsuitable buildings still in use' and the 'acute shortages of nursing and junior and medical staff' (ibid.). This speech provoked considerable discussion in the house and drew attention to some of the key problems facing psychiatry at the time. Forces for change were already in motion, however. In 1954, slightly before Robinson's speech, the Percy Committee was set up to look into the legal aspects of mental health. Its broad ranging recommendations, which formed the basis for the 1959 Mental Health Act, were published in 1957, by which time public concern about psychiatry had reached a considerable level.

We can get an idea of the way in which these issues surfaced in the wider public consciousness by considering some of the mental health stories from *The Times* for the year in which the Percy Committee reported: 1957. First, in February 1957, a negligence case was brought (unsuccessfully) before the High Court, concerning a man who had been 'crippled' as a consequence of ECT:

> On August 23, 1954, he was given a form of electrical treatment in the course of which, while he was unconscious, both of his thigh bones were forced through their sockets, which were smashed, and as a result he would never walk properly again.
>
> (*The Times* (Court Proceedings) 21 February 1957)

In July, this was rejoined by a debate in Parliament concerning the opening of inmates mail by staff (*The Times* 30 July 1957). Two stories in October illustrated further problems. First, a magistrate addressing a conference of the *Royal Society for Health* was quoted as saying that she and her fellow magistrates often felt 'guilty of manslaughter' on account of their role in the certification process:

> She declared: 'We hate it. We feel that we are in the hands of the medical officer. They often persuade us against our better judgement (Cries of 'Oh'). On a recent occasion I was called to help and certify an old lady of 90, and neither the medical officer nor I could find anything wrong with her at that moment. She answered all our questions. The

medical officer assured me that the only thing was certification because her daughter of 70 could no longer cope with her and was on the verge of a nervous breakdown.'

(*The Times* 19 October 1957)

Second, the provost of Sheffield, backed by the cathedral chapter and the *Council of Churches*, launched an attack on Sheffield's Regional Hospital Board. The provost pointed to the 'uncivilised' conditions at the city's 2089-bed mental hospital and to the failure of the board to act upon an earlier letter which he had sent to them:

> The Provost began the controversy by stating that a quarter of the hospital's patients slept in two vast wards, undressing on one floor and going up a stone staircase to the apparently unheated sleeping galleries. One ward had four lavatories for more than 100 patients and two of them did not work. There was no toilet paper. Another large ward had four wash basins with cold water only. At the time there were 100 cases of dysentery.
>
> (*The Times* 14 October 1957)

The publication of the Percy report, in May 1957, added impetus to this debate. *The Times* published a number of extracts from the evidence presented to Percy, which illustrated the extent of the abuses for example:

> ...after about eight years as a voluntary patient she asked to go home. She was given a paper to sign – she did not know what was in it – and was then sent to another hospital and certified.
>
> (*The Times* 31 May 1957)

> A woman referred to as Mrs D, who said that several years ago she spent a large part of a year in a mental hospital, complained of the 'regime of fear to which we were all subjected.' She said she was still in a state of terror that she might go into a mental hospital again.
>
> 'To the best of my knowledge I was never discharged as cured, although I was never insane all the time I was there', she added.
>
> (Ibid.)

Furthermore, a letter from Christopher Mayhew M.P. argued that legislation needed to go beyond the recommendations of the Percy Report as the latter completely failed to address problems of overcrowding, underfunding and dilapidated buildings (*The Times* 1 June 1957).

Much of the critique of mental health services within the field of psychiatric contention at this point in time was an overspill of official (parliamentary) processes of review and reform. Since at least the run up to the 1930 *Mental Treatment Act* the government had been concerned to reform mental health, removing, as far as possible, its custodial trappings and poor law associations (see Chapter 3), and refashioning it as a health service for ill people. By the 1950s, with the formation of the Percy Committee, they were warming up for another bout of reforms, which would culminate in the 1959 *Mental Health Act*, another major reform. This meant asking serious questions and that, in turn, took the lid off Pandora's box. More questions were asked than could be answered, more problems identified than could be solved. The inevitable result was 'social strain' and its occasional by-product, protest. Expectations were raised that could not be fulfilled, such that dissatisfaction began to find an outlet elsewhere.

The outcry provoked by these claims and revelations was in most cases relatively short-lived. They were, in effect, potential trigger events which failed to trigger any lasting or significant movement; sparks thrown up by the heat of strain which failed to catch on. That is, with the exception of the earlier trigger events concerning wrongful confinement, which were, as noted above, taken up by the NCCL. The NCCL campaign was only one of many at the time, as I have shown, but it was distinctive and significant because the NCCL framed its critique within the newly emerging discourse of civil rights, a discourse which was rising to prominence in the United States on account of the black civil rights movement. The civil rights discourse involved a relatively high degree of theoretical elaboration and linked the struggles within which it was invoked to fundamental values, thus lending those struggles a degree of gravitas and a sense of coherence. It was a discourse sufficient to sustain a social movement and, as just noted, it was linked with movement mobilisation in the United States. By comparison, the other critiques and campaigns of the time were little more than exclamations of dismay and horror. They lacked the discursive elaboration necessary to organised and sustained mobilisation. In addition, the NCCL was a pre-existing SMO, an organisation primed for sustained campaigning and looking for 'good causes' to adopt. It manifest 'mobilising structures' and it sought, as Zald and McCarthy's (1994) entrepreneurial model predicts, to 'supply' the 'demand' for change being expressed, or as Blumer (1969) suggests, to 'agitate' (see Chapter 2). For these reasons, the NCCL's campaign, though only one of many and not sustained into the 1960s, can be viewed as the first development of the birth of a new social movement within the field of psychiatric contention, alongside mental hygiene: a civil rights movement. Furthermore, though the involvement of the NCCL in this area, as noted earlier, did not last, the discourse of civil rights, once diffused into the field, remained. It had no representative SMO again until the 1970s but the discourse and frame became embedded.

A thorough analysis of this movement would have to trace the history of the NCCL (now *Liberty*), which I do not have the space to do. My analysis must rest upon the observations already made in this section. Namely: that reform of mental health services led to a rise in expectations which was quicker than actual changes in practice, a mismatch which resulted in strain and many potential trigger events. In many cases these events failed to trigger any sustained action, not least because there was no adequate framing of them, to focus and encourage activism. However, the emergence of the discourse of civil rights and of an SMO, the NCCL, formed around this discourse, provided the further ingredients necessary to carry grievance through to mobilisation and movement formation. They had both the framing and the organisational structure necessary to high profile protest.

The next key SMO to emerge as a representative of the civil rights movement/discourse was the NAMH itself, in the early 1970s. However their early response to this and the other critiques was not favourable. By the mid-1960s, a more critical stance is evident in their publications. An article published in their journal, *Mental Health*, in 1965, for example, argued that optimism about Community Care was rooted in 'wishful thinking', rather than facts (Jones 1965); and two further articles, in 1966, focused on cruelty and civil liberties in relation to the aged asylum population (*Mental Health* Summer 1965, 3–14). Notwithstanding this, however, NAMH were by no means at the vanguard of this critical edge and tended to assume the role of apologists for psychiatry, at least during the 1950s. When NCCL's *55000 Outside the Law*, was reviewed in *Mental Health* (1951, X(3), 80), for example, the reviewer was extremely cautious, prefacing most claims with qualifiers like 'alleged' and 'it is said'. The review questioned whether the 'as yet not proved' allegations had been taken 'somewhat out of proportion'. Indeed, the reviewer suggested that the existing problems could probably be accounted for by nursing shortages, a problem which s/he hoped would not be made worse by the negative publicity created by the pamphlet. Likewise, when the formation of the Percy Commission was discussed in an editorial of the journal, it was argued that patients didn't need protecting from doctors. The old legislation, it was claimed, was '... apparently designed to prevent victimisation by unscrupulous doctors – an attitude which is surely unnecessary today even if anyone supposes it was necessary 100 years ago' (*Mental Health* 1954, XIII(2), 50). In their presentation to the Percy commission, NAMH did acknowledge the importance of patients rights, but they were careful to put forward the other side of the story, arguing that the rights of the public, to be free of the nuisance and potential danger created by the mentally ill, should not be compromised. Moreover, the main part of their submission to the Percy Commission was framed by hygienist concerns, rather than civil rights matters.[4] This general position was echoed in the Parliamentary contributions of their chairman, Lord Feversham, both upon publication of the Percy Commission Report and the second reading of the 1959 *Mental Health Act* in the Lords. On the first occasion, discussing liberty, he argued:

> ... some machinery must exist for the welfare of patients who are unwilling to accept treatment, and for the protection of the community. The pendulum of public emotion swings dangerously between the

desire to lock up every potential murderer in a mental hospital and the belief, provoked by Press campaigns, that all hospitals should be emptied of patients, whether they be rightly or wrongly detained.

I would submit that the public need guidance on these matters.

(*Parliamentary Debates*
1957–58 (Vol. 2))

The reference to 'Press campaigns' in this quotation clearly indicates the distance which Feversham (who made clear that he was speaking as the chairman of NAMH) wished to put between himself and the civil rights lobby, and the reference to 'public guidance' reaffirms the paternalistic stance which NAMH assumed at the time. In his contribution to the second reading of the 1959 Bill, however, Feversham (again stating his position as chair of NAMH) made quite clear that he was in no position to offer such guidance. He would be concentrating upon how the Bill should be implemented rather than taking up the questions other Lords had raised regarding 'personal liberty', he argued, because there were men better qualified than he in the house to talk on such matters (*Parliamentary Debates* 1958–59 (Vol. 5)). In particular, demonstrating his deference towards and trust in the medical profession, even in relation to such non-medical matters as liberty and rights, he singled out two eminent doctors.

Guidance for the public was also a key theme in the book-length response which *Mental Health*'s editor, Tredgold, compiled in response to *The Plea for the Silent*. In his Introduction to the book, *Bridging the Gap*, Tredgold considered the charges levelled at psychiatry in *The Plea for the Silent* and related accounts. The extent of abuse was, he claimed, not as great as might be suggested by media reports and rumours. But lack of information and knowledge about psychology, psychiatry and the psychiatric system did create a great potential for problems and confusion. It was this confusion that *Bridging the Gap* aimed to address; the gap being bridged was between those who know and those who do not. The main body of the book thus comprised articles by mental health professionals which aimed to shed some light on the processes involved in mental health.

From the point of view of the longer history of psychiatry, mapped out in Chapter 3, there was little that was new in these debates. Even the intervention of the NCCL and the rallying cry of civil rights could be seen to mirror the earlier antagonism between medics and lunacy reformers (see Chapter 3). Even if this fresh wave of criticism was a 'return of the repressed', it was, however, a return and it was a fresh wave, following a period of relative calm in psychiatric politics. As such, it marked a transformation in the field of psychiatric contention – in particular the field became contentious again. The progressive agenda of mental hygiene began to take on a more conservative hue when its advocates found themselves defending the status quo within psychiatry against the criticism of outsiders, such as the NCCL, and indeed against such insiders as the contributors to

*The Plea for the Silent.* Indeed, it is arguable that the meaning of mental hygiene was transformed by the emergence of these new voices of critique, insofar as these new voices generated a new frame for public debate on mental health matters. No sooner had the central SMOs of the mental hygiene rescued themselves from potential crisis through amalgamation in the context of NAMH than a new crisis was impending, in the form of new, more critical actors in the field of contention. The critique in the 1950s was nothing compared to what would follow, however, as we see in Chapter 5.

## Conclusion

In this chapter I have sketched the history of the field of psychiatric contention between 1930 and 1960. During the earlier part of this period, the field was dominated by four SMOs (CAMW, NCMH, CGC and MACA), each of which embodied the discourse and represented the movement of mental hygiene. However, pressure generated by dynamics in the field led to the merger of three of them within the context of a new SMO: the *National Association of Mental Health*. Specific changes inducing this pressure included the formation of the welfare state, which was itself the result of dynamics and pressures in the wider societal field, including, but far from exclusively, the call of some hygienists for a professionalisation of welfare services, and the growing similarity and structural equivalence between the SMOs. The former tended to undermine the role of traditional voluntary sector organisations whereas the latter brought them increasingly into competition and conflict.

The *National Association of Mental Health* continued to embody and promote hygienist concerns throughout the 1950s, alongside the SMO which had refused to merge (*The Mental Aftercare Association* or MACA) and other smaller organisations. There was at least some tension here in the respect that MACA had rejected the merger on principle and thus embodied this difference of principle within itself, albeit a difference within the broader consensus constituting mental hygiene as a discourse and movement. A greater source of tension for NAMH, however, derived from the fresh wave of controversy and protest that was washing over psychiatry in the 1950s, controversy surrounding wrongful detention, mistreatment of patients and overcrowding in the mental hospitals – which, as I noted in Chapter 3, reached the peak in their population levels in 1954. Numerous trigger events were sparking localised conflict and protests. The strain underlying this protest and its conditions of conduciveness had derived, in part, from the elevation of expectations generated by the successive rounds of reform of psychiatry in the 1930s and 1950s and the tendency of these rounds of reform to open mental health practices up to question and criticism. And through the agency of the recently formed *National Council for Civil Liberties*, they were increasingly framed in terms of the discourse of civil rights, a discourse which was high on the political agenda across the Atlantic, where the black civil rights movement was gathering pace, and which was thus filtering its way into collective consciousness in the United Kingdom too. A new discourse and movement was establishing itself within the field of psychiatric contention: one based around civil rights.

The response of NAMH at this stage was to defend both psychiatry and the government, which they did by reducing critique to ignorance. The critics, they argued, failed to understand psychiatry, and they actually made things worse because one of the greatest threats to effectiveness in mental health services is public fear, which slows down the rate at which illness comes to the attention of psychiatrists and thereby increases the likelihood of chronicity. Listen to the experts NAMH pleaded, and, by way of a counter-protest, they stepped up their efforts to bring expert knowledge and opinion to the uninformed masses.

The final and important key point that I have attempted to bring into focus in this chapter concerns networks. NAMH, I have argued, were very well connected in a number of important respects. They were thus part of the establishment, with the various constraints and opportunities this presents. At the same time, however, they were in themselves a vast network, linking: (1) their own national, regional and local offices (2) various international mental health and related organisations (3) numerous national mental health related organisations and professional associations. If the field of psychiatric contention and indeed the wider mental health field was 'connected' then NAMH played no small part in bringing this about. It was a central hub where multiple lines of connection converged. This was no doubt significant in the 1950s, contributing to NAMH's status. It was also to prove significant later, as a mobilisation structure for more critical groups. That, however, is a topic for later chapters.

# 5 Anti-psychiatry and 'the Sixties'

In July 1967, four psychiatrists, one of whom, at least, described himself as an anti-psychiatrist (Cooper 1967), organised a two week long international congress at London's Roundhouse (the venue was taken over for the fortnight, with many of the younger participants electing to squat there for the duration). The congress was entitled *The Dialectics of Liberation* and its headline speakers included some of the key radical political thinkers and activists of the 1960s. Two of the conference organisers themselves fell into this category but other headline speakers included Herbert Marcuse, Allen Ginsberg, Lucien Goldmann, Paul Sweezy, Gregory Bateson and the leading voice of the US black power movement, Stokely Carmichael. Psychiatry and the political issues it raises were amongst the topics discussed at the congress but, as the line up suggests, there was also a much wider focus, incorporating a variety of what were perceived to be deep rooted structural problems of society and radical proposals for their resolution. Psychiatry had found itself on the agenda of the contentious politics of the 1960s. Indeed, in this particular case, psychiatry and psychiatrists or rather 'anti-psychiatrists' were at the centre of the contention; organising and agitating.

The four psychiatrists in questions went under the collective name of the *Institute of Phenomenological Studies* (IPS). Individually they were Ronald ('R.D.') Laing, David Cooper, Joseph Berke and Leon Redler. *The Dialectics of Liberation* was the best known of their collective projects, with the *Anti-University of London*,[1] instigated by Berke and Cooper, running a close second. However, in addition to the *Institute*, Laing and Cooper had also, four years earlier, co-founded a charitable organisation with five others,[2] *The Philadelphia Association* (PA). The PA, which by 1967 included Berke, Redler and their colleagues, Morton Schatzman and Jerome Liss, ran small therapeutic communities in London, the most famous of which was *Kingsley Hall* (open between 1965 and 1970). In its prime *Kingsley Hall* too was a central hub for the radicalism of the 1960s. It was a place where 'doctors' and 'patients' lived side by side but where, at least in theory, there was no organisational or symbolic distinction between them. Formal psychiatric diagnoses were not recognised. Indeed, they were rejected as harmful labels and, at least during the heyday of the community, the distress and mental disorganisation of those ordinarily on the receiving end of these labels was conceived as an 'existential voyage', a 'journey into inner space' which they should be allowed to pursue with the support of others and without the usual psychiatric interventions (Laing 1964b). The most famous 'traveller' from the community was Mary Barnes, an artist, whose trip involved a regression to earliest childhood; a state in which she could neither feed nor clean herself and was sometimes known to daub both herself and the walls of her room in her own excrement (Barnes and Berke 1973, Mullan 1995).

As with *The Dialectics of Liberation*, the remit of *Kingsley Hall* extended well beyond mental health. As Schatzman recalled, it was something of an educational establishment:

> The PA has sponsored lectures in psychiatry, 'anti-psychiatry' and phenomenology at Kingsley Hall, and has arranged seminars and professional meetings there with professional people in many fields... Experimental drama groups, avant-garde poets, artists, musicians, dancers and photographers, social scientists of the New Left, classes from the anti-university of London, and leaders of the commune movement have met at Kingsley Hall with the residents there in the last three and half years.
>
> (Schatzman 1969, 301)

For this amongst other reasons, it became a counter-cultural magnet; somewhere to see and be seen, even amongst those who were already well-known and fashionable figures. As Laing's son, Adrian, recalls:

> The reputation of Kingsley Hall spread with enormous energy. This was a place where one might find R.D Laing, Aaron Esterson, David Cooper on rare occasions, and definitely Mary Barnes – all under the same roof. There were no 'patients', no 'doctors', no white coats, there was no 'mental illness', no 'schizophrenia' and therefore no 'schizophrenics' – just people living together. The visitors became increasingly frequent and celebrated. Kenneth Tynan dropped in, as did David Mercer, Timothy Leary and Sean Connery. It was not uncommon for psychiatrists from all corners of the world to turn up ...
>
> There was a feeling of revolution about Kingsley Hall. The ideas and the people were so radical that the focal issues created the feeling that Kingsley Hall was a paradigm of psychiatric revolt, itself part of a wider, greater revolt, against the 'old order'. It was all terribly exciting.
>
> (Laing 1997, 108)

Word had got out about *Kingsley Hall* through the network channels of the counter-culture and 'underground'. And its notoriety continued even after it had closed, both by way of former PA member, Clancy Sigal's fictionalised critique, *Zone of the Interior* (a novel which Laing prevented the publication of in the United Kingdom) and more particularly by way of a joint account written by Mary Barnes and her chief PA therapist, Joseph Berke (Barnes and Berke 1973). The latter was taken up by leading playwright, David Edgar, and turned into a successful, widely and well-reviewed play.

These were by no means the only literary products of 'anti-psychiatry', however, nor indeed the only one's to be dramatised. A number of PA and IPS members published widely read and well-received books and articles, including Cooper, Berke, Esterson and Redler. They infiltrated and to some degree 'colonised' the reading publics of the liberal and new left, becoming 'required reading' within its social circles, and were at the top of reading lists for many university courses in the social sciences and humanities. It is no accident that Malcom Bradbury, building a picture of the radical protagonist of his campus novel, *The History Man*, by describing his room, identifies a book by Laing lying around. A book by Laing, at this point in time (the early 1970s), would have been as sure a sign of radicalism as a book by Marx or Trotsky, and would have been virtually *de rigueur* for a trendy lefty. As Peter Sedgwick, a critic of anti-psychiatry puts it:

> ... virtually the entire left and an enormous proportion of the liberal-arts and social-studies reading public was convinced that R.D. Laing and his band of colleagues had produced novel and essentially accurate renderings of what psychotic experience truly signified. Seldom can a vanguard minority of researchers, opposed to the orthodoxies of a dominant applied science, have achieved in so short a span of years a cultural or even political dominance of their own amongst progressive circles of the public with a pretension to discrimination in the matter of ideas.
>
> (Sedgwick 1982, 6)

As this quote and my own lead into it suggest, Laing was the 'star' of this band of 'movement intellectuals'. The members of the IPS and PA (the latter included all members of the former after a while) formed an inner circle of anti-psychiatry, at least initially, but it was Laing whose books were best-sellers throughout the world. In addition to the aforementioned Barnes–Berke collaboration, it was Laing whose ideas were turned into television and stage plays, who went on numerous international lecture tours through the late 1960s and 1970s, and who appeared regularly on British television and radio, even on such mainstream interview formats as the *Parkinson* show. And it was Laing who appeared on the front covers of all manner of popular magazines, including the trendy youth music magazine, *Melody Maker*. He was even to be found on mass produced car bumper stickers which bore the logo, 'I'm mad about R.D. Laing'. Even in the early 1980s, shortly before his death and long after the first wave of anti-psychiatry had peaked and declined as a cultural-political force, Laing could still draw a crowd. As one of my interviewees, an eminent professor of psychiatry who liked, respected and partially agreed with Laing, testified:

> ...when we had a meeting of Ronnie Laing at one of the [fortnightly public seminars on mental health issues] they actually called the fire brigade out because – we had it in the big lecture theatre in the medical school – so many people had come. They turned two or three hundred people away. They were sitting in the aisles, there was not a space. The police and the fire brigade said it was dangerous to have so many people.
>
> (Interview 1 (psychiatrist))

In this chapter I am going to trace the birth, heyday and eventual decline of this first wave of anti-psychiatry in the United Kingdom, a sharp departure from the genteel charity work of the *National Association for Mental Health*, discussed in Chapter 4. I will privilege Laing to some extent in this account, approaching the collective history of anti-psychiatry by way of his personal biographical history of involvement. This is justified by his centrality to the movement and is necessitated both by the relative wealth of information available about him and the dearth of information in relation to the other key protagonists. I will try, where possible, to make this the history of a collective, however. Moreover, I hope that even where this chapter is focused upon Laing, it remains a collective history. I mean two things by this. First, Laing, like anybody else, was not an isolated atom. His actions were inter-actions with others and his ideas were the products of dialogue, real or imagined, immediate or mediated, with others and with schools of thought which influenced and shaped him. Second, like a contemporary pop star Laing was, in some respects, a product of the publics who read and celebrated him; a point which is nicely captured in the distinction that Adrian Laing draws between 'Ronnie', the father he knew, and 'R.D. Laing', the public celebrity. R.D.'s influence and significance were not reducible to Ronnie as a flesh and blood individual. He was influential and significant to the extent that he was defined as such in the lifeworlds of the many who read and 'followed' him. I do not mean by this that he was a mere representation in radical culture. R.D. was one of Ronnie's roles and had to be played to exist. But by 'following' him his followers invested him with meaning, status and symbolic power, thereby positioning him to play that role in and for their movement. Moreover, their expectations and the pressure upon him to meet those expectations played an important role in shaping the role that was 'R.D. Laing', albeit in dialogue with Ronnie's own agency and input. In this respect 'R.D. Laing' was a social fact, a collective property.

The chapter contains four major sections. In the first, I briefly discuss the notion of 'anti-psychiatry' and the ideas associated with it. In the second I argue that anti-psychiatry emerged out of a failed 'scientific revolution' in psychiatry, in Kuhn's (1970) sense. In the third section, I consider the opportunity structures which facilitated the rise of anti-psychiatry, generated by the emergence of the new left, the counter-culture and the 1960s 'wave of contention' (see Chapter 1). These first three sections of the chapter effectively constitute my explanation of the rise of anti-psychiatry. In the final sections I step back from the historical and processual detail of anti-psychiatry, discussed in the main body of the chapter, in an effort to model its emergence theoretically.

In the next chapter I will link these developments in anti-psychiatry back to the material on NAMH and civil rights discussed in Chapter 4, and to a range of further movement currents. I will, in other words, situate anti-psychiatry within the field of psychiatric contention. It is impossible to do this without having first described and accounted for anti-psychiatry, however. I therefore ask the reader's forbearance. We will return to the central plot and idea of the book when this necessary and hopefully interesting digression has been properly explored.

## The anti-psychiatry movement?

Talk of 'anti-psychiatry' and of an anti-psychiatric movement immediately raises three problems. First, 'anti-psychiatry' was a label coined by Cooper (1967) and it is not clear whether the other members of the inner circle would have described themselves in this way. Certainly Laing disowned the label, claiming that he was never 'anti' psychiatry (Mullan 1995). Second, Laing also disputed the idea that there was an anti-psychiatry movement; in his view what many people referred to as a movement was, in fact, a handful of like-minded individuals (ibid.). Finally, the ideas of all of the members of the inner circle, but perhaps Laing in particular, shifted quite dramatically over time and, at some points at least, combined multiple elements in a way which seemed far from coherent, making them difficult to pin down to a single, coherent discourse, such as is suggested by the notion of an 'anti-psychiatry movement' (Sedgwick 1982). Furthermore, there were clearly disagreements and differences in emphasis between members of the inner circle. Is this chapter therefore based upon a false premise? Perhaps there never was an anti-psychiatry movement in the United Kingdom?

In response to the first of the above points note, first, that 'anti-psychiatry' was the label that stuck to the activities of Laing *et al.* in the 1960s and 1970s, whether they liked it or not. This alone justifies nominal use of it. Like all labels it simplifies and effects a classification on the basis of one or two of a multitude of properties and attributes, but like most labels it demarcates something of significance in relation to purposes at hand. In the case of this chapter it serves to demarcate the activities and ideas of a particular social network at a particular point in time, a network which became known, for better or for worse, as 'the anti-psychiatrists'. Second, the label 'anti-psychiatry' does not seem too far from the mark as a description of at least some of Laing's publications in the period that I focus upon here (1964–74). He was very critical of psychiatry and his critique extended to its role in contemporary society, its foundational categories and *raison d'être*. Psychiatry, he argued, is a mechanism of social control, necessary to the reproduction of an unjust and stultifying social order but not necessary in the wider schema of things and antithetic to the better world that he and other 1960s radicals aspired towards. This is not the kind of critique that would have been satisfied through a little tinkering with psychiatric practice. The changes it called for would have effectively transformed psychiatry beyond all recognition. Bearing this in mind, I think that Laing's hostility to the label 'anti-psychiatry' must be understood, in part, as an effect of him changing his mind about certain matters in the later 1970s and retrospectively altering his biographical narrative accordingly. In addition, considering both that Cooper invented the term and that the anti-psychiatrists became marked by splits and factions later in their collective career, there is perhaps some reason to believe that his repudiation of 'anti-psychiatry' was as much a strategy in the ego politics of the PA as anything else. Laing was hostile to the label 'anti-psychiatry' because it was Cooper's term and not his own – although there were genuine differences of opinion between Laing and Cooper.

An easy way out of the charge that anti-psychiatry was not a movement would be to quibble over what Laing understood by 'movement'. Does he mean what I mean by 'movement'? A more honest response, however, would be to concede that, at one level, anti-psychiatry was constituted by a relatively small nucleus; an 'inner circle' which spawned a number of SMOs with overlapping memberships: the PA, IPS and *Kingsley Hall*. However, as noted above, the impact of this nucleus, which had a steady in and outflow of members in the course of the late 1960s and early 1970s, was considerable and the diffusion of their ideas and sympathies extensive, such that the wider, more diffuse network of anti-psychiatry, a network constituted in some part by broadcast, publication and citation networks, was enormous. Moreover this was not simply a matter of excited reading publics who liked to read and talk 'anti-psychiatry'. Within mental health circles many psychiatrists, nurses, social workers and of course 'patients' were inspired to act differently, to alter their practices, as a consequence of anti-psychiatry. The psychiatrist, Anthony Clare, for example, claims that Laing '... influenced a whole generation of young men and women in their choice of psychiatry as a career', himself included (Clare 1992). And he adds that Laing's first book, *The Divided Self*, 'made an enormous impact upon me' (ibid.). Laing was encouraging young people into the mental health professions but was doing so on the basis of a very specific and unorthodox version of psychiatry. From the other side of the psychiatric relationship, Laing received thousands of letters from patients, many claiming that he, in contrast to their own psychiatrist, understood them (Clay 1996). Some even relayed this back to their psychiatrist. A number of psychiatrists, including one

I interviewed, who subsequently became friendly with Laing and an activist in various projects, took this positively:

> ...I think that I got very impressed with [Laing] because a lot of patients had read [*The Divided Self*] and I think that most psychiatrists were telling them not to and I was impressed by them saying 'he understands me, you don't'. The patients liked him.
>
> (Interview 1 (psychiatrist))

Others were less impressed, including the following contributors to *BJP*:

> Bright young schizophrenics, like bright young people generally, are interested in reading about their condition. From the vast and varied selection of literature available to them, they seem to show a marked preference for R.D. Laing's *The Politics of Experience* (1967). The present authors, like other members of the 'square' older generation, are of the opinion that they know what is best, and that this book is not good for these patients.
>
> (Siegler *et al.* 1969)

Amongst the changes in practice that this diffusion of ideas stimulated and shaped were a number of big projects, including attempts to build therapeutic communities like *Kingsley Hall*. Even where the changes were relatively small, however, they are significant and they are certainly sufficient to warrant talk of a 'movement'. Things were 'moving' in psychiatry, both in the sense of 'changing' and in the sense that new ideas and practices were passing through a network. In both cases this entailed that psychiatry, in some places and some respects, was being 'done' differently. Moreover, as noted earlier, the impact extended beyond mental health circles, into campus cultures, artistic and new left circles, to name only the most obvious. There may have been no mass marches on Parliament but there was clearly more to anti-psychiatry than a handful of disgruntled friends experimenting and getting things off their chests. The PA, IPS and *Kingsley Hall* were three amongst a number of anti-psychiatric SMOs, not all of which directly involved Laing, which serviced and drew from a much more extensive web of interest, enthusiasm and support for the evolving discourse(s) of anti-psychiatry and the projects which embodied them. The combination of this web and the SMOs which serviced it, amongst which I include the many artistic projects inspired by anti-psychiatry, amounts to an anti-psychiatry movement in my book.

The final criticism is far from damning. The ideas of Laing *et al.* varied, changed and were often not internally consistent. This applies to many social movements. We would have very few social movements in our analytical pot if our definition of them required that they speak with a unified voice in respect of a relatively unchanging discourse. Of course the lack of a single, unified ideology does make matters more complex. We have to be clear to specify, if possible, where in time and (social) space particular practices and ideas belong. But this only adds to the sense of a movement 'in movement'.

## A revolution in psychiatry

At the heyday of anti-psychiatry and even at the time of his first and (eventually[3]) most famous book, *The Divided Self*, Laing was based in London. He had a private practice as a recalcitrant and unorthodox but properly trained psychoanalyst[4]; he was a trained psychiatrist; he was a senior researcher at the Tavistock Institute of Human Relations, having previously worked as a senior registrar at the (separate but linked) Tavistock clinic to fund his training with the Institute of Psycho-Analysis; and he was director of the unorthodox Langham clinic, a nexus for psychiatrists, psychotherapists and psychologists with philosophical (particularly phenomenological and Eastern philosophical) interests. Laing was a Scot, however; a Glaswegian. He had trained as a medic in Glasgow (1945–51), had spent some time working in Stobhill hospital in Glasgow and then the nearby Killearn Neurosurgical Unit (both 1951). And following two years of national service in the Royal Army Medical Corp, which involved a number of postings (1951–53), had returned to work at the Gartnavel Hospital, the clinical base of the Glasgow Royal Mental Hospital (1953–55). This was followed by a brief posting at the Southern General Hospital, also in Glasgow (1955–56). It was only in 1956 that he moved south to undertake a psychoanalytic training at the Institute of Psycho-Analysis.

During this early period Laing acquired first hand experience of both military and NHS psychiatry, and performed the normal tasks of a junior psychiatrist. He had begun to write and research, however, even as a medical student, and many of the themes of his later 'anti-psychiatric' work are evident in this very early work, albeit, and significantly, framed differently. In his very first published paper, 'Philosophy and Medicine', for example, he argued that medicine should be more informed by philosophy because the latter could furnish it with important concepts, addressing the nature of human beings, which it had not and arguably could not produce for itself. This argument is the first airing of a claim that would be developed throughout his early work; namely, that psychiatry needs to engage with the whole, situated person, the person as being-in-the-world, as explored in existential phenomenology.

This argument and indeed the arguments in all of Laing's early work, up to and including the first editions of both *The Divided Self* and *Self and Others*, are innovative and Laing recognised them as such but they are not presented as challenges to conventional psychiatry, nor are they completely out of step with the psychiatry of the day. Philosophy was a marginal interest in psychiatric circles but it was a legitimate interest and some medics were prepared to take it seriously, as the reviews of Laing's early work attests. *Self and Others* was reviewed in both *The Lancet* and *BMJ*, for example, and both reviewers found something positive in it:

> The book is difficult but peculiarly fascinating in that it enables the reader to share what may be termed the poetic insight of a scientifically educated mind. If the psychiatrists neglect it, the novelists will not.
>
> (*The Lancet* 7 July 1962)

> Some of its theories, such as that of the breakdown of the self by non-confirmation through other people, may appear fanciful, yet this theory is closely akin to the hypothesis that schizophrenic breakdown may be caused by sensory deprivation, an aspect of the subject which is being assiduously studied by physiological methods today. Though most psychiatrists will find the author's approach uncongenial and unhelpful, therapeutically, they will recognise and even defend it as one possible way of viewing and describing mental disorder.
>
> (*BMJ* 19 May 1962)

For his own part, Laing was always at pains to emphasise that his interventions were limited in scope and were intended as positive contributions to psychiatry rather than negative critiques of it. In an early paper on Paul Tillich's work, for example, he argues that

> Tillich is not interested in making a destructively critical attack on our theories based upon clinical experience, but rather to contribute to their clarification. We must all agree that the basic assumptions of our work are not as explicit as we would like them to be. Tillich believes that such clarification must come from an awareness of our ontological assumptions about man.
>
> (Laing 1957, 88)

Laing clearly identifies himself as a psychiatrist amongst psychiatrists in this passage, referring to 'our theories', 'our work', what 'we must like' and what 'we must all agree'. He also clearly takes the sting out of any negative critique that might be discerned in his advocacy of Tillich's position by proleptically disclaiming the notion that Tillich is a critic. Tillich, he insists, is not making a destructive attack and therefore, by implication, neither is he. Likewise, in the *Preface* to the first edition of *The Divided Self*, which would later become a sacred text of anti-psychiatry, Laing is careful to frame his discourse as a very partial venture which advances on marginal fronts that psychiatry has neglected. He is not, he explains, rejecting the central tenets of psychiatric science, nor is he seeking to compete with them. They lie beyond the scope of his altogether more limited project:

> ...no attempt is made to present a comprehensive account of schizo-phrenia. No attempt is made to explore constitutional or organic aspects. No attempt is made to describe my own relationship with these patients, or my own method of therapy.
>
> (Laing 1961, 9)

Exactly why Laing pursued these marginal avenues is a more complex question. Certainly the explanation relates back to his early education. On the positive side, he had been educated at a grammar school which specialised in classics and humanities and, inspired by this, he had taken very early in life to reading philosophy; becoming particularly interested in Kierkegaard and then later Heidegger and Sartre but remaining open to many schools and always taking philosophy as a standard bearer of truth (Clay 1996). This passion for and commitment to philosophy in his early life is revealed in a number of instances in his biography, not least by the fact that he formed his own philo-sophical debating forum whilst at university, 'The Socratic Club', inviting Bertrand Russell to be its president (Russell accepted) (ibid.). Negatively, the humanities emphasis in his formative education was at the expense of a full scientific education (ibid.). Furthermore, unlike many medical students of the day his parents were not medics (he was from a lower middle-class back-ground). Whether or not this affected his competence to compete on the scientific terrain with his contemporaries in psychiatry is an open question – he did fail his final year examinations in medical school and admitted that he found the scientific basis of medicine difficult to learn – but I suggest that it did mean that he approached medicine and psychiatry as an outsider. He was not disposed, through early inculcation, to 'believe in the game' to quite the extent that some of his contemporaries were. Given these peculiarities in his educational career, we might interpret his early philosophical interventions in psychiatry as consisting in three aspects. First, he had learned to enjoy philos-ophy and find it meaningful but he had not had the same formative experience in relationship to science, and he was therefore simply following his 'heart' and doing what interested him. Second, as an outsider to medicine and the scientific worldview he was disposed to see its shortcomings, a disposition reinforced by the critical questioning encouraged in philosophy. As an insider to philosophy, moreover, he was disposed to see 'urgent' philosophical ques-tions in the psychiatric enterprise, questions which had to be answered before psychiatry could move on. His psychiatric colleagues, of course, might have argued that he was too enmeshed in the game of philosophy to notice its short-comings and insufficiently enmeshed in theirs to grasp its urgent matters. From this point of view his actions might be regarded as an expression of his sense of duty. He was trying to do what was right and best, as he saw it. He was pursuing the truth. It is important to add here that, philosophy aside,

Laing appears to have been moved by a genuine sense that the 'mentally ill' are people in distress, behaving meaningfully. He could not reduce them to 'patients', as clinical practice demanded, nor to 'biological machines', as biochemical science demanded, and the appeal of existential-phenomenology to him was undoubtedly amplified by the fact that it offered an alternative to these reductions. He wasn't merely pursuing what he believed to be true, in this respect, but also what he believed to be right; recognising the other as a person. Finally, given that competition for dominance in the psychiatric field was tight and that he enjoyed both a relative wealth of philosophical capital and a relative lack of scientific capital, we might interpret his actions strategically, as an attempt to play to his strengths and carve out a niche for himself. I lack any data that would allow me to decide between these interpretations but in any case I suspect that the proper explanation for Laing's action involves elements of each. There is plenty of evidence from Laing's biography that he was ambitious and strategic but there is also plenty of evidence that he was passionate about both philosophy and people. I would thus suggest that Laing pursued a philosophical path in psychiatry, early in his career, because he loved philosophy, believed that it raised essential issues for psychiatry and could see that he was in a strong position to play this card and accrue whatever benefits doing so might bring.

Laing's early interventions were not restricted to philosophy, however. In an early paper in *The Lancet* he discussed an experiment that he and his colleagues conducted at Gartnavel, which effectively prefigured *Kingsley Hall* and the other therapeutic communities of the PA (Cameron *et al.* 1955). In what was colloquially known as 'the rumpus room' traditional nursing practice had been abandoned in an effort to generate a more communicative, positive social environment for chronically ill patients. The results, Laing *et al.* reported, were positive (ibid.). Significant improvements in the mental health of the patients were recorded. This work clearly overlaps with his philosophical preoccupations, in the respect that the existential-phenomenological theories he was interested in hinged upon issues of intersubjectivity and the relation of self to other.

Similarly, his early work at the Tavistock Institute was focused upon patterns of interaction, particularly within the family. He devised a method for the analysis of family interactions (Laing *et al.* 1966), for example, and, with Aaron Esterson, embarked upon a major study of patterns of interaction within the families of schizophrenic adolescents – the unfulfilled aim of the project as a whole was to compare these with patterns in 'normal' families. Later this study, whose initial findings (on the 'schizophrenic' families) were published as *Sanity, Madness and the Family* (Laing and Esterson 1964), would be framed by Laing and his commentators as a critique of the family. Laing frames its findings very differently at different points in his biography, always flagging his current interpretation as an index of his original intentions. However, it is clear that the studies for *Sanity, Madness and the Family* were intended, like the 'Rumpus Room', Laing's early philosophy and the methodology proposed in *Interpersonal Perception*, as serious contributions to psychiatry as a scientifically based discipline. The rhetoric is certainly scientific, referring to experiments, controls, results, etc. Furthermore, as with the philosophy, the aims of the project are stated in quite modest terms. Laing and Esterson do not claim to be challenging psychiatry. Nor do they claim to be exploring the causes of 'mental illness'. The primary purpose of their investigations, they claim, is to allow us to better understand mental distress by seeing it in its context.

These studies were not out of step with other work in psychiatry at the time. Psychiatry was, then as now, relatively eclectic, even if, then as now, biology tended to predominate as the foundational discourse within this eclectic mix. The 'Rumpus Room', for example, was one of a number of similar projects and experiments being tried out at the Gartnavel Hospital in Glasgow, where Laing was based between 1953 and 1956, some of which pre-dated Laing's arrival at the hospital. In addition, as noted in Chapter 3, psychiatrists had been experimenting with 'therapeutic communities' and interaction patterns ever since they had first encountered shell shocked soldiers during the First World War – the respective works of Maxwell Jones and Wilfred Bion, both of which Laing could be expected to be familiar with, had made these issues relatively high profile in UK psychiatry. The Tavistock Clinic, where Laing was first employed upon moving to London, was a key site of practice in this respect; a centre of social psychological and therapeutic innovation. On the other side of the Atlantic, moreover, the work of the anthropologist, Gregory Bateson, and the 'Palo Alto School' of family therapists to which he was attached, were exploring similar themes, and achieving some critical acclaim.

The timeliness of Laing's work is further illustrated by the fact that the year he published the first edition of *The Divided Self*, 1961, Thomas Szasz published *The Myth of Mental Illness*, Erving Goffman published *Asylums* (both in the United States) and, in France, Michel Foucault published *Histoire de la Folie* (his second critical book on madness). Both Szasz and Goffman, like Bateson, situated the behaviour of the mad within a context of social interaction, and both, along with Foucault, were considerably more critical of psychiatry than Laing had been up to this point. Indeed, as noted, the latter wasn't particularly critical at this time.

The timing of much of the above-cited work is too close to make any strong claims with regard to lines of influence. Moreover, philosophically at least, each came from a rather different direction. By the mid 1960s, however, Laing had become aware of the work of Bateson, Szasz and Goffman, at least, and was beginning to pull them together in the context of his own work. In his opinion these ideas were revolutionary. The revolution he had in mind was not political, however, nor was it 'anti' psychiatry. He summed up his position in the conclusion to an article in *New Society* in 1964:

> I have given a glimpse of a revolution that is going on in relation to sanity and madness, both inside and outside psychiatry. Modern psychiatry came into being when the demonological point of view gave

way 300 years ago to a clinical view-point. The clinical point of view is now giving way before another point of view that is both existential and social. The shift, I believe, is of no less radical significance.

(Laing 1964a, 17)

There is a striking parallel here with Szasz (1972), who opens *The Myth of Mental Illness* with a quote from Karl Popper: 'Science must begin with myths, and with the criticism of myths' (1957, 177). In both cases the critique of psychiatry and the suggested path forward are presented as an advance within psychiatry, an advance which will further enhance its scientificity and efficacy. This is not a revolt against psychiatry but rather what Thomas Kuhn (1970) was later to refer to as a 'scientific revolution'. Where Kuhn is agnostic with respect to claims about progress, however, Laing and Szasz, perhaps in closer conformity to Bachelard's (1970) ideas on 'epistemological breaks', believe that this revolution marks a genuine step forward for psychiatry. The rhetoric of scientific progress is clear and unequivocal. Laing framed his new views as progress *within* psychiatry, a psychiatric revolution rather than an anti-psychiatric revolution.

The fact that writers such as Goffman, Bateson and Szasz were arriving at similar conclusions to him, independently both of him and of each other, undoubtedly served to bolster Laing's sense that he was right and that the time for these new ideas had come. Moreover, these distant sources of confirmation were complemented by more immediate and direct sources. The Tavistock Clinic was a central hub in the UK network of psychotherapists and humanistic social scientists. Furthermore, Laing had become involved in the 'Open Way' (later renamed the Langham Clinic), a meeting place for therapists with an interest in phenomenology and Eastern philosophy which, Adrian Laing claims, 'had a magnetic effect on the intellectuals around at the time' (1997, 65). By way of these two sources Laing had begun to meet like-minded people and to test out and disseminate his ideas. He had circulated drafts of *The Divided Self* prior to publication, for example, and had given seminars on his work at the Open Way. He was achieving support and recognition. Others within his immediate environment were listening to him and agreeing. Moreover, the networks that would give birth to both the PA and IPS were beginning to take shape and Laing was emerging as a central player in these networks. His main collaborative work can be dated to this time. In 1958, for example, he met David Cooper, a South African psychiatrist who had moved to London and was, when they met, working at the Belmont Hospital. Cooper was always much more of a 'big P' political thinker than Laing, more drawn to Marxism and to various oppositional ('anti') projects. The two shared a passion for Sartre, however, which resulted in a collaborative book, *Reason and Violence*, in 1964. *Reason and Violence* was an exposition and discussion of Sartre's later work, *Critique de la Raison Dialectique*. Moreover, Cooper also shared an interest with Laing in therapeutic communities. In 1962, when working at Shenley hospital, he set up his own experimental community, *Villa 21*.

Like Laing's *Rumpus Room, Villa 21*, which was open until 1965, was a precursor of *Kingsley Hall*, slightly overlapping in time with it.

Cooper was involved in the PA and *Kingsley Hall*, as was another collaborator of this time, Aaron Esterson, whose first-hand experience of the Kibbutz in Israel provided his credentials and motivation for experimental forms of living and caring. Esterson and Laing had met as students at Glasgow University and had written together as early as 1958. In the early 1960s, however, Esterson too moved to the Tavistock and began work with Laing on the abovementioned study of interaction patterns in families of schizophrenics.

The connections and expressed support multiplied as these collaborative works, particularly *Sanity, Madness and the Family*, began to attract attention outside of Laing's immediate circle, and even in the national media. Laing made his first, relatively low key TV appearances in 1963, and embarked upon his first US lecture tour in 1964. This tour brought him into face-to-face contact with a group of four young American medical students who were later to move to the United Kingdom, join the PA and become centrally involved in *Kingsley Hall*: Joseph Berke, Morton Schatzman, Leon Redler and Jerome Liss (Berke 1969). All were excited by his ideas.

It is little wonder, considering this supportive reference group mirroring back confirmation to him, that Laing believed the collective effervescence he was living through to be a scientific revolution. As Kuhn (1970) recognised, however, scientific revolutions are always necessarily political revolutions too, in the respect that they challenge the authority and legitimacy of an old guard who have invested a great deal in the existing paradigm and who, in virtue of this, are both too deeply enmeshed in it to recognise the need for change and are inclined to fend off attacks from 'upstarts' who challenge their position. It is the fate of many challenges to dominant paradigms to fall on deaf ears and find themselves 'nipped in the bud'. And this is what happened to the innovations of Laing *et al.*, at least as far as their reception in the psychiatric and wider medical field was concerned. Even those who sympathised with Laing's ideas, at least if they enjoyed any degree of investment in the psychiatric field, found it very difficult to become his fellow travellers to the extent that revolution requires. As one of my interviewees, who was head of a Medical Research Council research unit at the time, explained:

> ... it also struck me that the politics of research was very much influenced by the fact that, however much I was thinking like that, if I changed direction everyone would lose their jobs. Because then, you know, they backed the director of the unit, the research unit and everyone had complicated contracts.
>
> (Interview 1 (psychiatrist))

At a more direct level, however, Laing was finding his ideas blocked. Most mainstream psychiatrists were not impressed by his ideas or tended to see them as interesting asides to the real business of psychiatry. Moreover, as Laing upped the ante, challenging the orthodoxy more directly and positing his own approach as an alternative, he met increased resistance. Clay's (1996) biography suggest that an article Laing wrote in 1962, criticising the genetic theories of schizophrenia which were rising to dominance at the time, proved a critical turning point. It was turned down by four journals including the *British Journal of Psychiatry* (*BJP*) and the Tavistock's own in-house journal. John Bowlby, at the Tavistock, was concerned that the paper was too polemical and not clinical enough. It was not unusual for Laing's articles to be rejected by the *BJP* (Mullan 1995, 355) but rejection by the Tavi indicates that Laing's trajectory and that of conventional psychiatry were pulling in different directions. He was approaching a fork in the road.

## Straddling ships: the new left, the counter-culture and the cycle of contention

It was time to sink or swim. He either had to conform to the demands of the psychiatric field or find another field in which to 'play'. In effect he chose and was chosen by the latter. On one hand his growing popularity and celebrity as an author and psycho-commentator were providing outlets for him. He didn't need medical journals to communicate his ideas. More importantly, however, changes in the nature of left wing politics and the social circles attached to it, in particular the rise of the 'new left', combined with the wave of contention and rise of the counter-culture in the 1960s, were creating new audiences, publics and opportunities. This point needs to be unpacked.

The narrow focus on economics that had characterised left wing politics in the United Kingdom prior to the 1960s was giving way. New left con-stituencies were increasingly interested in questions of philosophy, culture, health and the politics of such 'superstructural' formations as gender, the family and health/welfare services. This change in direction was marked by, amongst other things, the launch of the *New Left Review* in 1960. Laing *et al.* had numerous connections to the social circles of the new left, at least in London, and they also fitted neatly into this new social space, being in a position to 'supply' what was demanded. In particular Laing's work on Sartre and on family dynamics struck a chord. Thus, as publication opportunities in psychiatric journals were closing down, opportunities in political journals were opening up. Laing *et al.* were able to jump, or at least straddle, ships.

The move away from psychiatry and towards the new left, which was never absolute, is illustrated nicely in the pattern of Laing's journal publi-cations. It is clear from Table 5.1 that Laing did not cease completely to publish in medical journals in the 1960s but there was a marked shift in his publishing pattern. He begins to publish in social (*New Society*) and political (*New Left Review*) journals.

Table 5.1  Laing's early and later journal papers

| Year of Publication | Title of article | Title of journal |
|---|---|---|
| 1949 | Philosophy and Medicine | *Surgo* |
| 1950 | Health and Society | *Surgo* |
| 1953 | An Instance of the Ganser Syndrome | *Journal of the Royal Army Medical Corps* |
| 1955 | Patient and Nurse | *The Lancet* |
| 1957 | An Examination of Tillich's Theory of Anxiety and Neurosis | *British Journal of Medical Psychology* |
| 1958 | The Collusive Functioning of Pairing in Analytic Groups | *British Journal of Medical Psychology* |
| 1962 | Series and Nexus in the Family | *New Left Review* |
| 1964 | What is Schizophrenia? | *New Left Review* |
| 1964 | Is Schizophrenia a Disease? | *International Journal of Social Psychiatry* |
| 1964 | Schizophrenia and the Family | *New Society* |
| 1965 | Results of Family Oriented Therapy with Hospitalised Schizophrenics | *British Medical Journal* |

It is not only the place of publication that was beginning to shift, however. So too was his tone and both the inferences he was drawing from his ideas and the way in which he was framing them. We see this even in the contrast between his two *New Left Review* articles. The first sought to apply two key concepts from Sartre's *Critique de la Raison Dialectique*, 'series' and 'nexus', to the study of the family. The *Critique* was the culmination of Sartre's conversion to Marxism. As such, Laing's application might be regarded as inherently 'political'. Aside from 'guilt by association', both in terms of outlet and influence, however, there was nothing particularly political or critical about the article. Laing was not 'coming out' as a Marxist or any kind of political critic. The article posited a further exploration of the family dynamics that had always interested him, by way of the new work of a philosopher whose work, similarly, he had a longstanding interest in and passion for.

The second article, in 1964, was a different kettle of fish. In this article he explicitly attacked the psychiatric establishment. Psychiatrists, he argued, are 'so possessed' by their belief in an 'entirely hypothetical pathological process' that they have ceased to recognise it as hypothetical. Furthermore, assumedly referring in part to his own unpublished paper, he argued that recent critiques of genetic explanations had brought the discipline back to square one. There was no basis to psychiatric categories or ideas, he claimed. This much might be reconcilable with a scientific revolution, just about, but the article went further. What we call 'psychosis' or 'schizophrenia', he argued, is an 'inner voyage', a journey into 'inner space', but in contrast to our fascination with outer space, manifest at the time in the 'space race', we close ourselves off from inner space and seek to control those who are inclined to journey within it. We label them negatively and sequester them. Referring to the labelling process, he suggests researching a new mental illness, 'psychiatrosis'. Moreover, in a section entitled 'A Political Event' he criticises the controlling function of psychiatry and proclaims:

> I do not myself believe that there is any such 'condition' as 'schizophrenia'. Yet the label is a social fact. Indeed, this label as social fact, is a *political event*. This political event, occurring in the civic order of society, imposes definitions and consequences on the labelled person.
>
> (Laing 1964b, 64)

Later in the paragraph Laing spelled out exactly what he believed these consequences were:

> After being subjected to a degredational ceremonial known as a psychiatric examination he is bereft of his civil liberties in being imprisoned in a total institution known as a 'mental hospital'. More completely, more radically than anywhere else in our society he is invalidated as a human being.
>
> (Ibid.)

And he outlined the implications of this view for the future of his own work:

> ...this work must now move to further understanding, not only of the internal disturbed and disturbing patterns of communication within families, of the double-binding procedures, the pseudo-mutuality, of what I have called the mystifications and untenable positions, but also the meaning of all of this within the context of the civic order of society, that is, of the *political* order, of the ways persons exercise control and power over one another.
>
> (Ibid., 65)

The sources that Laing refers implicitly to here are much the same as in his abovementioned 'scientific revolution' paper. They are Bateson and Goffman. But the framing has completely changed. Processes which were once conceived, for the most part, as interpersonal or familial are now conceived as social and political, and are connected with a broader conception, albeit vague and unexplicated, of the social and political order. Furthermore, the interactions and relationships comprising the family have shifted from being a context which gives meaning to the words and experiences of its distressed members and, at most, a hypothetical factor in the aetiology of this distress, to being a site of 'disturbed and disturbing patterns of communication', 'double-binding procedures', 'pseudo mutuality' and 'untenable positions'. This is now a critique, simultaneously clinical and political, of the family, and Laing is effectively doing what he criticises other psychiatrists for doing; affording hypotheses (regarding the role of the family in relation to mental distress) the status of established truth. For its part psychiatry has shifted from its subject position, as a 'we' who might address these issues, to an object position, as the thing or issue being addressed. Though, to a large extent, Laing is addressing the same problems he had been addressing for some time, these are no longer framed as problems for psychiatry to examine but rather problems with psychiatry that an external (to psychiatry) social critic should be alert to.

When *The Divided Self* was reissued in 1965, it too was reframed. I noted earlier that Laing was careful in the *Preface* to the first edition of the book to take any sting out of the material he was presenting. He emphasised the very partial and complementary nature of the exercise he was conducting. The preface to the second edition was rather different. He begins by disclaiming aspects of the book by reference to his age at the time of writing it and (assumedly) his political innocence:

> One cannot say everything at once. I wrote this book when I was twenty eight. ... This was the work of an old young man. If I am older I am also now younger.

The book has the merit of examining madness in its context, he argues, and of examining the power situation in the family (which may be true but the term 'power' is not used in either edition, with the exception of this prefatory remark) but it falls into a trap: 'I am still writing this book too much about Them [i.e. mental patients] and too little of Us [i.e. the people who deem mental patients mad and lock them up].' This comment is followed, firstly, by reference to the repressive nature of civilisation and 'one dimensional men', thus keying in to the work of the leading 1960s radical, Herbert Marcuse (1986, 1987), who would later speak at the *Dialectics of Liberation* congress and who's *One-Dimensional Man* Laing had reviewed in *New Left Review* in 1964. Second, by a challenge to the conventional distinction between sanity and madness which, in turn, was keyed in to one of the most controversial political issues of the day, the cold war and the threat of nuclear annihilation:

> ... a little girl of seventeen in a mental hospital told me she was terrified because the Atom bomb was inside her. That is a delusion. The statesmen of the world who boast and threaten that they have Doomsday weapons are far more dangerous and far more estranged from 'reality' than many people on whom the label 'psychotic' is affixed.
>
> (Laing 1965, Preface)

Moreover, he once again turned upon psychiatry:

> Psychiatry could be, and some psychiatrists are, on the side of transcendence, of genuine freedom, and of human growth. But psychiatry

can so easily be a technique of brainwashing, of inducing behaviour that is adjusted, by (preferably) non-injurious torture. In the best places, where straightjackets are abolished, doors are unlocked, leucotomies largely forgone, these can be replaced by more subtle lobotomies and tranquilisers that place the bars of Bedlam and the locked doors inside the patient. Thus I would wish to emphasise that our 'normal', 'adjusted' state is too often the abdication of ecstasy, the betrayal of our true potentialities, that many of us are only too successful in acquiring a false self to adapt to false realities.

(Ibid.)

The false self described in the book is thus no longer identified exclusively, if at all, with the neurotic or psychotic individual. The 'well-adjusted' individual whom psychiatry takes as an ideal is no less false, on account of the crazy world to which they are well adjusted. Indeed they are more false.

The new left was by no means the only audience or public for such claims. This was the 1960s and Britain, like most other Western democracies, was in the early stages of a wave of contention. A culture of protest was spreading, particularly on university campuses, and both the number of political groups in society and their respective levels of activity were increasing. In addition, what became known as the counter-culture was beginning to take shape; a culture of opposition to the *status quo* and of experimentation with new and novel practices that went well beyond the politics of the new left.

There has been much nostalgic mythmaking about the 'counter-culture'. There is good sociological evidence of strong changes in both the attitudes and practices of young people through the course of the 1960s, however. The work of Musgrove (1964, 1974) is an interesting case in point. Having conducted a survey of youth attitudes and activities in the early 1960s, Musgrove found himself publishing his results at a point where those very attitudes and activities seemed to be undergoing a profound transformation (Musgrove 1964). Consequently he set about replicating his own study almost immediately, and what he found offered strong support for the idea of a counter-cultural wave of change (Musgrove 1974). Ideas and more particularly the practices of everyday life for young people had changed markedly. They were stepping outside of the norms and roles previously expected of them, collectively effecting change through the excited and experimental interactions that Durkheim (1915) dubs 'collective effervescence'.[5]

Musgrove's study dates the key period of change between 1964 and 1969. This makes Laing an 'early riser' and opinion leader of the counter-cultural current. Moreover, his links to the counter-culture, and those of his circle, ran deep. At one level there is no doubt that the counter-culture and its personalities fascinated him and drew him in. He was eager to connect with the 'stars' of the movement and took advantage of a lecture trip in 1964 to meet both Timothy Leary and Allen Ginsberg. There were also many interesting overlaps between the counter-culture and Laing's own innovations in psychiatry, however, which served as bridges he could cross and investments he could capitalise upon. His examination of family inter-actions and their relationship to mental distress, combined with his interest in therapeutic communities, for example, resonated with counter-cultural opposition to parental authority and the family, as well as the counter-cultural embrace and idealisation of communes as an alternative family form. In addition, like a number of psychiatrists of the time he had been experimenting, from the very early 1960s, with the therapeutic potential of LSD. The drug was of interest to psychiatrists, in large part, because certain of its effects mirrored certain of the symptoms of psychosis, but for Laing it seemed to have the further benefit of facilitating the 'inner journeys' that were of such therapeutic interest to him. An LSD trip was akin to the free association practiced in conventional psychoanalysis or indeed to the dream, which Freud describes as 'the royal road to the unconscious'; a way to peek behind the defences of the psyche. Within a few years he had estab-lished himself, at least within his social circle, as something of an expert on LSD, and had done so quite independently of the counter-culture. This res-onated with the counter-cultural profile of LSD and other mind-altering drugs, however, allowing him, later, to occupy a position akin to that of Timothy Leary in the United States. He became an oracle to consult on drug matters, particularly in relation to the problem of 'bad trips'. One 1960s rebel, for example, describes a situation in which his girlfriend had a bad trip and he, thinking she may be dying, took her to the only person he thought could help: 'Ronnie was helping her. The Man. I'd taken her to the Man. I went and lay on the bed and in the end it was the greatest trip I ever took.' (Marcuson, cited in Green 1988). Beyond this, moreover, Laing had a track record as a philosopher of alienation, love, self-development and personal relations; he was a critic of science and technology. All of this stemmed from his 'legitimate' academic studies, studies he had once tried to make acceptable to the psychiatric establishment, but they resonated strongly with the themes of the counter-culture and therein acquired a new framing, meaning and value. With a little tweaking Laing had the perfect CV for a hippy guru. Somewhat paradoxically his status as a medical doctor, a member of the establishment, did not seem to count against him here. Indeed, as far as one can tell it counted for him. He was important because he had all the credentials of an establishment figure but seemed to turn back on the establishment and to use the expertise it had given him against it. R.D. Laing questions the distinction between madness and san-ity, dismissing schizophrenia as a socio-political label, and he should know, he is a psychiatrist! R.D. Laing, a doctor, experiments with LSD. He'd hardly do that if there was any danger, and again he should know as he is a doctor. And so on. He was just enough of an establishment figure, with sufficient establishment credentials, to be a star of the anti-establishment.

Of course these bridges could only be made if Laing was prepared to reframe his ideas and interests. We have already seen that he was. Indeed,

Laing went further than reframing. He began to incorporate elements of the counter-culture into his writings. The abovementioned references to the atomic bomb, the definition of psychiatric diagnosis as a political act and the references to power and civil liberties all bear witness to this. Moreover, much of his later writing manifested a further departure still from the psychiatric game. In 1967, with the publication of *The Politics of Experience*, his polemic and critical approach reached its zenith. *The Politics of Experience*, a summation of the political themes and theories he had been developing in the three of four years preceding it, also manifest a shift towards a more flow-of-consciousness style of writing, however, and the simultaneously published *Bird of Paradise* marked a shift towards a poetic style of writing that was to remain the dominant style in Laing's work thereafter. Whole books were written in poetic form. To get a flavour consider the following extracts from *Knots*, first published in 1970:

> They are playing a game. They are playing at not
> playing a game. If I show them I see they are, I
> shall break the rules and they will punish me.
> I must play their game, of not seeing I see the game.
> (Laing 1971a, 1)

> She has started to drink
> as a way to cope
> that makes her less able to cope
> the more she drinks
> the more frightened she is of becoming a drunkard
> (Ibid., 29)

*Knots* was a best-seller in many countries on both sides of the Atlantic and, like a number of the earlier works, was adapted for stage. It is fairly obvious, however, that Laing had abandoned any attempt to make an impression in the psychiatric field. All of the basics of academic discourse, let alone medical discourse, had been ejected. Laing does not offer arguments, evidence or even continuous prose. He communicates to us now poetically, by means of allusion. The twists and turns, the 'knots' and contradictions he finds embodied in human relations manifest directly in the twists and turns of his poetic verse. This is not the way to impress and persuade medics. It departs radically from medicine's language game and positions Laing closer to the beat poets than to psychiatry.

It is also interesting to note, in this connection, the phrasing of the above-mentioned disclaimer Laing uses in the second edition of *The Divided Self*: 'This was the work of an old young man. If I am older I am also now younger.' Although it is impossible to prove a direct line of influence, there is an intriguing echo here of the Bob Dylan song, *My Back Pages*, which first appeared on the album, *Another Side of Bob Dylan*, in 1964, one year before Laing's new *Preface* was published.[6] Each verse of *My Back Pages* ends:

> Ah, but I was so much older then,
> I'm younger than that now.

If Laing has borrowed from Dylan – and it looks to me as though he has, given that this is an unusual and distinctive turn of phrase – this would again show the extent to which the counter-culture was permeating his work, and would tend to reinforce the idea that this permeation was a significant factor shaping the transformation of progressive psychiatry into anti-psychiatry.

Laing wasn't the only member of the inner circle who was writing, however, and writing wasn't the only practice engaged in by the anti-psychiatrists. After Laing, Cooper was perhaps the most widely read of the anti-psychiatrists. His best known work, published in 1967, was a book which gave the movement its name: *Psychiatry and Anti-Psychiatry* (Cooper 1967). As noted earlier, Cooper was generally more political than Laing, more wedded to Marxism and more oppositional. This is evident in *Psychiatry and Anti-Psychiatry*, a book which outlines his philosophy and describes the experiment in *Villa 21* – a description which plays with scientific language and is described as ironic but which nevertheless betrays Cooper's own attempt to straddle the psychiatric and counter-cultural worlds. Furthermore, Cooper followed the project through in the 1970s, publishing a scathing attack on the family (*The Death of the Family*) and further work on madness (*The Language of Madness*) as well as more philosophically oriented works (*The Grammar of Living*). Esterson, in contrast to Cooper, was less political and critical than Laing, but he developed his own publishing career and reputation, notably with a study which extended the existential and interactionist studies that he and Laing had begun (*The Leaves of Spring*). Likewise there were publications by Berke, Schatzman and Redler.

Beyond publication, as noted at the outset of this chapter, were such projects as the *Dialectics of Liberation*, the *Anti-University of London* and the various therapeutic communities of the PA, chiefly but not exclusively *Kingsley Hall* (the PA ran nine houses a different times through the late 1960s and the 1970s). The former two of these projects clearly grew out of counter-cultural environment that facilitated the emergence of anti-psychiatry, and they demonstrate the desire and ability of the anti-psychiatrists to take a leading role within it. As far as I can tell Laing was not directly involved in the *Anti-University*. That was a project initiated by Berke and Cooper – though *Kingsley Hall* played host to some of the classes, so Laing would have been 'around'. Laing was involved in the *Dialectics*, however, which was the bigger of the two events, being defined by some commentators as one of the central events of 'the 1960s' (see Green 1988). Certainly it passed into legend, the 'counter-memory' of the 'counter-culture', and indeed into vinyl and film. LP records of the speeches were pressed and several documentary films recorded (Laing 1997).

*Kingsley Hall* was different, being more directly tied to the psychiatric aspect of anti-psychiatry. It was central to the movement too, however, constituting what I have referred to elsewhere as a 'working utopia' (Crossley 1999b). Working utopias appear in many social movement contexts. They are spaces where the aspirations of the movement appear, to some degree, to have been realised. As such they serve a variety of purposes, some intended, others unintended, for the movement. They serve as 'laboratories', where new ideas can be tested out and their problems ironed out; as 'schools', attracting interested parties who, through involvement, learn to do these new practices and carry them out into the wider world. They excite and energise activists, symbolising the feasibility of the hoped for future and lending meaning to struggle by embodying the dream. Moreover, as this excitement exerts a magnetic draw upon activists and would-be activists, pulling them together in a contained time–space, they help to generate the networks that effective social movements presuppose. They are social capital generators. In addition, for activists they constitute 'proof' of the veracity of critiques and proposed alternatives. Though, of course, critics watch them closely in the hope of them providing refutations. All of these aspects can be seen in relation to *Kingsley Hall*. I have already noted the magnetic pull of the place and, by implication, its role in generating social networks. *Kingsley Hall* was a place to be and, as a consequence, a place where one met others who needed to be at the place to be. Part of its attraction, moreover, lay in both its experimental and its pedagogic value. Although a fashionable place to be seen amongst counter-culturalists it equally had an intrinsic interest to (politically and scientifically) progressive psychiatrists who wanted to see for themselves how such radical transformations of practice worked out in practice and to learn the lessons of the experiment. The pioneer of Italian democratic psychiatry, Franco Basaglia, who we will encounter later in this book, visited *Kingsley Hall*, along with other therapeutic communities in the United Kingdom, for just this reason. He is just one relatively famous example of a trend, however. Beyond this, *Kingsley Hall* was a central image in the collective imagination of many progressives and critics in the mental health arena, a 'promised land' where things really were better, and outside of the imagination it was, for different parties to the debate, both proof and refutation of the possibilities of doing mental health care in a better way.

### The subsidence

The fate of anti-psychiatry, or more specifically the energy, critique, controversy and imagination it generated, can only be assessed against the history of later developments that I will discuss in subsequent chapters. For now it must suffice to note that the bubble had burst by the early 1970s.

Tensions within the PA motivated some members, led by Berke, to form a breakaway group in 1970, the *Arbours Association*, and Laing enjoyed an uneasy relationship with those who remained, at least until he was effectively ousted in 1981. Moreover, the rise to prominence of other members of the inner circle and their 'growing apart' inevitably generated tension. Laing was no longer the sole voice. Esterson, Berke and particularly Cooper were competing for his audience, and also with each other. Moreover, each had a different vision such that ego clashes were mixed with struggles for symbolic dominance even within the inner circle. Esterson was more moderate than Laing, for example, and sought to further explore existential and interactional issues. Cooper, by contrast, was more radical, declaring 'death' to the family and psychiatry, and aligning himself with a more Marxist position.

The latter half of 1971 and first half of 1972 mark something of a watershed for this first wave of radical mental health activism. During this time, Laing took a year out in India and Sri Lanka to pursue his interest in meditation and Eastern religion/philosophy. Upon his return he reconnected with the PA and continued to write, lecture and provoke controversy. However, he had peaked, and his career as both a psychiatrist and a guru was in decline. He died in 1989, having been struck off the medical register in 1987 because he was deemed unfit to practice.

Other members of the inner circle remained active in the 1970s and Cooper in particular was peripherally involved with a number of developments which would become further important waves of activism (see Chapters 6 and 7). By the mid-1970s, however, the original project was beginning to wane. The PA and *Arbours Association* had both become more conventional and acceptable; Laing and Cooper, always the stars of the movement, had lost their shine; and the world had moved on.

### Paradigm shift?

Laing *et al.* had made a difference. Psychiatry would never be quite the same. Assumptions once questioned do not, at least immediately, sink back into place; and questioning and critique can become an institution. Having asked questions, formed networks and forged identities around a project, agents do not happily return to the *status quo ante*. Nobody had stormed the premises of the *Royal College of Psychiatrists*, blown up ECT machines or terrorised psycho-pharmaceutical companies. But the hopes, expectations and practices of a sufficient number of people had been changed to say that anti-psychiatry had exerted an influence. At the very least it had laid the seeds for further challenges, which I will discuss later in the book.

In terms of mainstream psychiatry the anti-psychiatrists did not achieve the paradigm shift that they had initially believed they would usher in. However, I believe that, at the very least, they prepared the way for a paradigm shift in the wider campaigning culture, the field of psychiatric contention, which revolves around mainstream psychiatry. I will discuss the reaction of the NAMH to anti-psychiatry in the next chapter. Suffice it to say, however, that their discourse on mental hygiene (see Chapter 4) looked decidedly dated and out of touch after anti-psychiatry. Psychiatric publics had, in a decade, been radically transformed. This was not only as a consequence of anti-psychiatry and of course nobody was forced to agree with anti-psychiatry. Most medics did not. But nobody could carry on as before after anti-psychiatry. The field of psychiatric contention was opened up for new, more critical trains of thought. The ground had moved and the paradigm shifted.

## Explaining anti-psychiatry: a concluding discussion

Hitherto in this chapter, I have tried to 'tell the story' of anti-psychiatry, giving a processual account of the way in which it unfolded and gathered steam. In this final section I want to step back from the fray, reworking the material already discussed in an effort to offer a more abstract account of the rise of the movement, focusing specifically upon the value-added model of movement formation discussed in Chapter 2. That model, I noted, identifies six preconditions for movement formation: (1) structural conduciveness (2) structural strain (3) discursive formation and diffusion (4) mobilising structures (5) trigger events and (6) the actions of third parties. How does this apply to anti-psychiatry?

The strains precipitating the rise of anti-psychiatry might be thought to derive primarily from the hardships experienced by patients. If we focus upon Laing, however, then this situation is complicated by strains he personally experienced in trying to change psychiatry. There can be no doubt that he felt compassionate towards the people he treated, that he tried to understand them and that his attempt to reform psychiatry was informed by this empathy and compassion. It was mingled with his own philosophical and interactionist interests, however, and it was the frustration of being unable to introduce the changes he desired which really generated the strain which, in turn, generated anti-psychiatry. Laing had raised expectations about what might happen in psychiatry, not least his own expectations, and it was the failure of these expectations to be realised which generated an impetus to rebellion.

The psychiatric field itself was not particularly conducive to struggle, at least in the early 1960s. This didn't really matter, however, as Laing had ample opportunities to make his case in the context of a transformed 'new' left, a growing counter-culture, a rising 'wave of contention' and a more general atmosphere of rebellion and opening up that was 'the 1960s'. The times, as Bob Dylan noted, were changing and as such they could not really have been better for a group of psychiatric rebels. This is a matter of opportunities but also more than that. In Zald and McCarthy's (1994) terms, Laing *et al.* supplied what the counter-culture was demanding. They stepped onto a stage that was calling out for performers and they played up to their audience, giving it what it wanted. A growing concern about the treatment of mental patients, their civil rights and the state of mental hospitals within 'straight society' (see Chapter 4) only contributed further to this.

In terms of discourse, Laing *et al.* were active producers and disseminators. Anti-psychiatry was a very popular new discourse in some social circles. However, it is clear from what I have argued in this chapter that the anti-psychiatrists absorbed a great deal from other critical discourses in play at the time, from phenomenology, Sartre and Marcuse through to Bob Dylan. In addition they benefited from the pre-existence of critical publics ready to receive their 'sort' of ideas. Without *New Left Review*, *New Society* and the readership these journals assembled anti-psychiatric discourse may have struggled to achieve the level of diffusion that it did. And of course these journals only had an audience on account of earlier journals and wider social movements. There was a discursive formation, in the full Foucauldian sense of an apparatus for producing and disseminating discourse, that Laing *et al.* were able to connect to, and this apparatus gave them a position from which to speak and be heard (Foucault 1972). However, the anti-psychiatrists did produce a new, hybrid discourse and it was a discourse which 'spoke' to many people both within and outside of psychiatry, resonating with a pre-existing sense of disaffection and alienation. This discourse, insofar as it framed and organised that disaffection, was a key element in the movement of anti-psychiatry.

Resources were not a problem. *Kingsley Hall* was secured for a nominal rent. It was effectively free, as were the other early communal properties. Given that all residents in these communities, doctors and patients alike, were expected to pay for their own keep, this meant that this branch of anti-psychiatric practice was without significant costs – although Adrian Laing records that his father was often in conflict with other members of the PA towards the end of his association with them as they wanted to engage in conventional forms of fund raising to expand and maintain activities whereas he rejected such 'establishment' methods. Given that the other activities of the anti-psychiatrists were not particularly cost-incurring, and that the inner core were all doctors, there were few financial obstacles to be overcome and the flow of resources, whilst essential to mobilisation, here as everywhere else, did not affect its timing.

Similarly, mobilisation structures did not pose much of a problem. The PA formed, first, out of a network of therapists and fellow travellers who met by way of their mutual involvement in innovative therapeutic and phenomenological projects in London, largely centred upon the Langham clinic. And then second by the addition of four college friends from the United States, some of whom met Laing on his first US speaking tour and all of whom eventually arrived at *Kingsley Hall*. By all accounts the 'management' of the organisation and its communities was sometimes chaotic and acrimonious but the group was always small so this didn't really matter. And the PA itself was quite well networked within the various circles of the new left and counter-culture in London, such that its members had easy access to these other channels. It is not perfectly clear from my research why and how these networks were formed, except to say both that *Kingsley Hall* was a counter-cultural magnet and that Laing, a 'natural networker', became very active in discussion fora upon arriving in the capital, which put him in contact with many people. Laing *et al.* were well connected in the new left and counter-culture and this undoubtedly helped. For example, Laing had connections with Perry Anderson, the editor of *New Left Review*, whilst Cooper was in a relationship with Juliet Mitchell, then an up and coming feminist/new left writer. Such informal links must have helped secure the place of anti-psychiatry within the circles of the new left, again without any cynical intent on behalf of anybody involved.

It is difficult to identify a single trigger event which set off the movement. The emphasis which Laing's biographers place upon the rejection of his critique of genetics by medical journals, combined with his own reference to it in his second *New Left Review* paper, suggest that this may have been a turning point for him, but the processual account offered in this chapter belies any notion of a single trigger event. The career and biographies of movements, like those of individuals, are perhaps best considered in terms of successive and cumulative 'turning points' generated through the coincidence of factors, both internal and external, to the gathering momentum of the collective.

As for third parties, media and broadcast networks were clearly a factor in carrying the ideas, practices and project of Laing *et al.* beyond a narrow psychotherapeutic clique, particularly the 'oppositional' media of both the new left and counter-culture. These 'underground' channels, as noted earlier, relayed anti-psychiatry to an audience who identified with it and took it as their own. The mainstream media helped too, of course, but their interest and that of their audience were, by definition, less attuned to the radicalism of anti-psychiatry. Beyond the media it is not clear that other external agents, played much of a role in the construction of anti-psychiatry. Run-ins with the police were minor as most of what happened was either within the law or at least no more outside of it than everything else connected to the counter-culture. However, the psychiatric establishment arguably played a key role. In blocking and sidelining the claims of the anti-psychiatrists, before they became 'anti-psychiatry', they arguably played the key role in provoking the attack they were subsequently subject to. If the psychiatric establishment had accepted Laing and his ideas there may never have been an anti-psychiatry movement in the United Kingdom.

# 6 Parents, people and a radical change of MIND

Although anti-psychiatry peaked, in terms of the activity level and profile of its key protagonists, in the late 1960s and early 1970s, declining after that point, its influence was considerable. It provoked a variety of different reactions and generated a range of effects in the field of psychiatric contention. And these reactions and effects, which carried some of the energy and controversy of anti-psychiatry, had their own effects, forming part of a chain reaction that is still running at my time of writing. It is these impacts and chain reactions, in part, which justify talk of a 'field' of psychiatric contention. They require that we focus not upon individual SMOs or even movements but upon the space generated by interactions by a range of such SMOs and movements, interactions which shape the identities and dispositions of their participants. This is not to say that anti-psychiatry was a prime mover or that it was the only influence upon subsequent developments in psychiatric politics. As we have already seen, anti-psychiatry was shaped by prior and external factors. And as we shall see, many factors have influenced the subsequent direction of psychiatric contention. But anti-psychiatry was very significant and in both this and Chapters 7 and 8 I will be seeking, amongst other things, to trace its lines of influence, seeing how they interconnected with other conditioning influences.

This chapter sets the ball rolling with an examination of three central developments in the field of psychiatric contention during the 1970s: (1) the first key development of what might be regarded as a backlash against anti-psychiatry, a 'counter-movement' which sought to challenge 'liberalism' in psychiatry (2) a radical transformation of the NAMH (see Chapter 4), which resulted in the growth of a strong civil rights perspective in the field of contention and (3) a spin-off of anti-psychiatry which intersects with both the *Mental Patients' Union* (discussed in Chapter 7) and the transformation of NAMH. I begin with this latter development.

## People not psychiatry

In 1969, two years after Laing's radicalism had peaked, with the publication of *The Politics of Experience*, a new radical network, initially called

*People for a New Psychiatry* but then later renamed *People Not Psychiatry* (PNP), began to take shape. Its original cell was based in London but as further cells began to proliferate within the capital they also spread beyond it. By 1970 there were cells in Leeds, Manchester, Birmingham, Glasgow, Edinburgh, Worthing, Brighton, Nottingham, Bristol, Cardiff, Stoke and Hull, to name a few. The idea behind PNP was to provide a network of contacts for individuals who were experiencing mental distress, who would offer them an alternative option to psychiatry and the mental hospital. The contacts in the network might, for example, talk the individual through their difficulties or they might offer material support, including a place to crash. PNP eschewed hierarchy and formal organisation. The network was a living organism which developed in accordance with the improvisation and initiative of all who were involved in it, each acting as they saw fit. As Jack, an early activist put it: 'There is no one that you have go to ask permission. You just tell people you are doing something' (Jack undated, 8). The network, Jack continues, is a resource that all of its members can use to develop their own initiatives, whilst simultaneously, by means of their initiatives, they enrich and replenish it. Above all, according to the network's founder member, Michael Barnett (1973), PNP was an experiment, an attempt to see if things could be done differently and in a better, more humane way.

For many members of the network notions of therapy, treatment or a professional relationship (between counsellor and counselled) were anathema. The focus was, as the group's name suggests, *people* rather than *psychiatry*. *People* were helping other *people*. And in many cases there was reciprocity; each side needed help and was prepared to help the other. Jack again:

> ...the important thing about PNP is that the people are not professionals. My role in PNP is not as a professional. And as soon as you pay me, give me a pad and support me for being a PNP person I'm no longer just somebody in PNP, another person. I've got a role; that makes me different from other people...
>
> (Jack undated, 10)

This is good for Jack, in the respect that he can help when he feels able to, leaving others to pick up the work when he is not. He does not have the responsibility or the obligations of a professional. But it is good, PNP documents insist, for those on the receiving end too because they get help from somebody like them, who understands and who is helping because they want to help – not because they are getting paid. The scope for help is unbounded in a way that professional help, shaped by job descriptions and the (understandable) competing demands upon professional carers, is not.

The 'crash pads' of the organisation were, in some cases, individuals' houses or flats. Some PNP activists were involved in other aspects of the 1960s, 'alternative scene', however, including squatting groups, such that squats too soon became available. Interestingly PNP's first squat was provided courtesy of Dr Robin Farquharson, acting as secretary of the *Situationist Housing Association* (SHA). Farquharson also later found a squat for the *Mental Patients' Union* (MPU) (see Chapter 7) and was involved in both organisations. PNP's founder member, Michael Barnet, was invited to join the committee of the SHA, which he did, along with Farquharson and Leon Redler, of Laing's inner circle and the PA. The aim of the SHA, according to Barnett, paraphrasing Farquharson, was to 'get a house like Kingsley Hall except that it will also having people living in it who are not currently agonising and who can act as helpers' (Barnett 1973, 191–2).

Barnett had a history of anti-psychiatric involvements prior to PNP. Having experienced mental problems of his own, his original inspiration was Laing. Speaking of *Self and Others* he writes,

> I sat down and began to read it, and it slowly began to dawn upon me that I had found home. Here was the definitive field, for it was about *me*, and it was about *others*, whom I had studied in my sly, subtle, avid, unavowed way for so long....I wrote the author congratulating him...but putting him straight on one or two points....
>
> (Ibid., 53)

Barnett followed this up by reading several of Laing's other works, including *The Divided Self* and *The Politics of Experience*, before deciding that he 'would have to go and see R.D.Laing' (ibid., 55). He paid for a session with Laing but was ambivalent about the counsel he received and annoyed that Laing stuck to the medical protocol of working through his (Barnett's) GP, talking about Barnett rather than too him. Following a recommendation from a friend and distant relative he therefore checked out two other members of the PA, Leon Redler and Aaron Esterson (whose books he had also read). Both proved more conducive. Indeed, Esterson used his influence to get Barnett a job as a nurse at a local, 'progressive' hospital, whose wards were modelled along the lines of a therapeutic community. Through Esterson he retained contact with the PA and got to know other members. He hovered around the inner circle.

The next step in Barnett's anti-psychiatric career was sparked by an article in *The Guardian* newspaper.

> I read of a new group with the picturesque name of Campaign Against Psychiatric Attrocities, or CAPA, that had been demonstrating outside a hospital against the use of neuro-surgery there. It touched my own latent fury. I rang the organiser, Peter Stumbke. He came to see me. He felt I could be of some use to him so we started working together at once....CAPA demonstrated further, and I marched with the rest, bearing my banner, 'Psychiatry Kills'.
>
> (Ibid., 73)

Barnett worked intensely with CAPA (not to be confused with the *Campaign Against Psychiatric Oppression*, CAPO, who I discuss in Chapter 8), over a number of months. He claims to have always felt slightly dissociated from the group and disconcerted at the lack of knowledge regarding the 'classical arguments' of anti-psychiatry among its key members, including Stumbke: 'He appeared to know little about Szasz and Cooper and Laing' (ibid., 77). Greater disillusion was to follow, however. The trigger was a visit to CAPA by PA member, Sid Briskin.

> Sidney sat there under my gaze and said, 'I hear CAPA is connected with Scientology.' I replied at once, brisk and business-like: 'Nonsense, no connection at all.' I became aware I was speaking alone; I had expected a chorus. I shot a look at Peter. He was still...I sensed disquiet. Briskin went on, a gentle executioner, 'I understand you at least have been a Scientologist for a number of years.' I was shattered to hear Peter confirm this. He went on, saying that CAPA was a separate, personal affair, but already I was lying numb against the ruins. I heard Sidney, far off, remarking on the coincidence that Scientology was currently mounting a mammoth campaign against psychiatry.
>
> (Ibid., 79)

I will return to Scientology's campaign against psychiatry later in the chapter. For the moment suffice it to say that this shock motivated Barnett both to leave CAPA and to make his own way in the world of anti-psychiatry: 'The time had come to toddle, to take my first steps alone.' (ibid., 81). He wrote a brief article in the underground journal, *International Times*, criticising psychiatry and announcing the emergence of a new group, *People for a New Psychiatry*. Establishing what would become a trademark of PNP, the article gave contact details for interested parties, of which there were several hundred. From amongst these Barnett selected 14 who, along with himself and his wife, would form the original core of PNP. These developments merited a mention in a rather more 'above ground' newssheet, which further spread the word.

> A difference of opinion has emerged amongst the militant opponents of modern psychiatry. Since March a group calling themselves the Campaign Against Psychiatric Atrocities have demonstrated in Harley Street four or five times, waving placards with slogans such as 'Psychiatry Kills' and 'Psychiatry Does You In'. Now Mr Mike Barnett, who was for a time the campaign's acting secretary, has left to organise a new movement – 'not a protest, but a positive alternative...'
> ...Stumbke says his parting with Barnett was amicable – 'A difference over methods not aims' – but Barnett seems to have been also concerned at the backing the campaign was receiving from the scientologists (whose enmity towards psychiatry has been manifested in

recent publications). Stumbke, however, denies that his campaign has any links with scientology.

(*The Times* 11 August 1969)

*People for a New Psychiatry* became *People Not Psychiatry* and, aided by contacts in the underground information network (BIT), its philosophy began to spread, generating a proliferation of cells nationwide. Underground and leftist journals seized upon this new innovation, interviewing activists, reporting developments and always accompanying such reports with contact details. Interested parties around the country were therefore able to connect with the original cell and add their contact details to the list, allowing the nodes in the network to proliferate. Moreover, when various members of any cell moved or spent time 'out of town' they took the message and the organising principles of PNP with them, fostering new groups in the locales they visited. PNP were in business, spreading and growing. Meanwhile, in London the original PNP cell, which had now recruited David Cooper and Clancy Sigal from the PA, had established a regular Friday meeting which became, in underground circles, a 'main event', particularly when another alternative network rising to ascendancy at the time, $P^2$ (that is, P-squared),[1] elected to hold their meetings at the same time and place. Like the anti-psychiatrists before them, PNP were connecting both with psychiatry and the counter-culture (some members were also involved in far left groups), and they were thereby bridging the two domains, informing radicals and counter-culturalists of the problems in psychiatry whilst simultaneously informing disaffected constituencies within psychiatry of the possibilities for protest and change opening up within radical and counter-cultural circles.

By the definition of Melucci (1989, 1996), PNP were a textbook 'new social movement' cell. Melucci describes how new social movements work to carve out alternative and experimental social spaces where new forms of identity and social practice can be tried out, new ways of living explored. This is just what PNP were doing. *Kingsley Hall* and the other PA houses fit this model too, of course, but what was really significant about the PNP network was its size. The practical activities of the PA and the IPS were inevitably limited by the fact that they were always a small group of close associates. Thousands of people were influenced by the activities of the PA and IPS but with the exception of a few who gained access to the inner circle, their connection to their influence was a weak, one-way connection; adherents were a readership and audience for Laing, albeit an audience sometimes mobilised by the words of the master(s). PNP was very different. It was vast by comparison, much less insular, inherently involving and thereby generative of connections and structure. Proliferation and involvement were essential elements of its philosophy. Individuals and groups were invited to 'connect' to it, adding their contact details and thereby contacting with and becoming a part of it. Barnett's claim that the network achieved 10,000 members strikes me as questionable but it was clearly large and sprawling.

Moreover, PNP challenged psychiatry in the decentralised and innovative ways characteristic of new social movements. It sought to lessen individuals' dependence upon the formal channels of psychiatry by providing an alternative to it, thereby striking at the heart of psychiatric power. The power of psychiatry rests in part upon the fact that distressed individuals and their families need help. 'Symptoms' are frightening and difficult to cope with for everybody concerned. Insofar as psychiatry has a monopoly on providing solutions for these problems, it is clearly in a very strong position. Of course psychiatry needs patients too. There is a relationship of interdependence between psychiatrists, patients and their families and friends. But the balance of dependence tips in favour of the psychiatrist, such that the balance of power, to borrow Elias' (1979) definition, does too. At least it does if distressed individuals have nowhere else to turn. When individuals construct alternatives to official services, in the form of crash houses and support networks, however, providing that these alternatives suffice both to meet their needs and to allow them to avoid the public forms of social deviance that constitute 'step one' of a psychiatric career (Goffman 1961, Scheff 1984), they lessen their dependence upon psychiatry and thereby shift the balance of power in their favour. When and where it is successful, this is a very effective challenge to psychiatry.

## Accounting for PNP

The founding 'spark' for PNP was Barnett's article in the *International Times*. His call to arms resonated with readers of the journal, moving them to contact him and thus allowing the first nodes of the network to fall into place. All of the indications are that those who became involved, who would have represented only a fraction of the *International Times*' readership, had a prior interest in psychiatry. They had experienced the 'strains' generated by psychiatry, such that what Barnett said was not new to them but rather a persuasive way of framing grievances they had expressed and felt themselves. The conditions of their involvement had been brewing, biographically, for some time. Indeed, Jack (undated) claims that most of the early participants, like himself and Barnett, had prior interests in anti-psychiatry, so they were prepared twice over for involvement; once by strain and once by adherence to the ideas and critiques of Laing *et al*. This discursive connection makes PNP an anti-psychiatric SMO by my definition (see Chapter 1) and also allows us to regard its formation, to some degree, as an effect of that movement. However, as readers of the *International Times*, PNP members were also pre-selected for involvement on the grounds of their wider radical and counter-cultural interests. The journal was a pre-existing broadcast network for the radically inclined, a mobilising structure that Barnett was able to plug into in an effort to generate support.

Barnett's article was thus a moment in a value-added process. It added the spark, the frame and the calling, but its success depended upon pre-existing strains, discourses and mobilising structures. And, of course, Barnett's own biography was as much shaped by these factors as the biographies of those he mobilised.

Structural conduciveness was also important, on four counts. First, PNP presupposed the existence of individuals who were experiencing mental problems in a context sufficiently free from constraint that they could pursue alternatives to psychiatry. For reasons I discuss later, mobilisation was very difficult in the hospital context. Even if the post-1930s hospitals were less custodial (Chapter 3) they were still constraining in a manner not conducive to activism. It was much easier for outpatients and day patients to mobilise, and mobilisation was therefore far more likely at this point in time (the 1960s), when the shift towards day and outpatient services had begun to kick in (Chapter 3). Second, within some circles at least, antipsychiatry had transformed cultural representations of mental problems in a way that made it easier for people to talk openly about them. The stigma attached to mental health problems was lifted, affording a space for those affected to be more inventive in their strategies for dealing with it. Indeed, echoing earlier days, when 'nerves' had been a rather fashionable complaint amongst the British middle classes (Porter 1987a, Scull 1993), mental problems could be framed in ways which lent their 'host' a sense of both radicalism and depth. Third, anti-psychiatry had made psychiatry perceptibly more vulnerable to attack, putting it on the back foot and generating resources (e.g. critical discourses) with which to attack it. Finally, antipsychiatry itself was only one element in a much larger wave of contention which involved a broad attack upon many of the key institutions of modern society. This wave opened doors and generated resources. It gave birth to the squatting organisations who provided PNP with crash houses. It gave birth to radical publications and related mobilising structures, which disseminated PNP ideas and allowed connections to be formed. Moreover, it was the crucible within which a new generation of political activists formed itself, a generation who were receptive to PNP ideas.

In terms of the final element of my value-added model, 'third parties', mainstream journalists played a part in the respect that their coverage of PNP circulated its ideas and raised its profile, helping the network to grow and spread. Beyond this, however, the greatest contribution of a range of agents who might have become involved, perhaps seeking to control PNP activism (e.g. medical and welfare agencies), was that they did not become involved, at least not to any significant degree. Obstacles which might have been thrown down were not.

As a final point on PNP, note that it was very closely connected both with CAPA, for whom Barnett had been secretary, and with various members of the inner circle of the PA. Barnett had visited Laing, formed a friendship with Esterson (who had got him a job) and Redler (who was on the committee of the SHA with him). It was Briskin who first alerted him that CAPA were scientologists. And both Cooper and Sigal were involved in PNP, to the point of regularly attending the Friday night meetings of the original cell. To this we must also reiterate the link with Robin Farquharson, the secretary of the SHA, who later provided a squat for the MPU (see later). The significance of these links is twofold. First, if we spot similarities between the various groups and projects discussed in this and other chapters we should not be surprised. When the people involved are not the same they are often connected. They meet, discuss and exchange ideas and resources. Second, and more importantly, the world of radical mental health politics, at this time, was a 'small world' and our focus of attention should perhaps be this world as a whole rather than the specific SMOs within it. Though it does not always apply, it is striking at certain points in the history I am recounting that named groups are little more than placeholders for the activities of a particular, temporary cluster within a bigger, constantly evolving network. Named groups come and go, sometimes rapidly, and often have vague and permeable boundaries, but the network to which they belong is a constant factor. The tangle around PNP, the PA, CAPA and even the MPU (who I discuss in Chapter 7) is one example of this. There are degrees of separation between them but there is also a great deal of overlap and interconnection. We would be ill advised to regard them as completely distinct SMOs and the picture falls more easily into place if we conceptualise them as overlapping regions of an underlying network that is more fundamental than them. Moreover, this wider network constitutes a central mobilizing structure for the various SMOs and projects that emerge within its mesh. With this said, we can turn to the next strand of the seventies developments; the radicalization of the NAMH.

## NAMH, anti-psychiatry and scientology

Anti-psychiatry did not receive a great deal of attention in the pages of NAMH's journal, *Mental Health*. Interestingly, however, when the texts of Laing, Goffman, Scheff and others were reviewed they generally received an open-minded and thoughtful response. NAMH reviewers were not about to 'tune in' or 'drop out'. There is no evidence that they identified with the counter-cultural aspect of anti-psychiatry. But they identified points they could agree with in these texts. This is not surprising since, as noted in Chapter 5, these texts, for all their radicalism, were radicalised reinterpretations of ideas which psychiatrists in the 'eclectic' British tradition had been toying with prior to the rise of anti-psychiatry, ideas akin to those advocated by the mental hygienists in NAMH. The idea that mental distress had social (and familial) causes, for example, was very much in tune with the claims of the mental hygienists. And the idea of group therapy and therapeutic communities, given a radical spin by the anti-psychiatrists, had been pursued in a more conservative and paternalistic fashion by NAMH itself.

Indeed, even when more radical, the claims of anti-psychiatry found some support from the contributors to *Mental Health*. When David Mercer's controversial, Laing-inspired television play 'In Two Minds' was first broadcast in 1967, attracting considerable criticism in the media and from psychiatrists, for example, *Mental Health* afforded Mercer a full article to reply to his critics. Their own review of his play stated that, although controversial, it had provoked interesting and useful debate (*Mental Health* Summer 1967).

NAMH's recognition of Laing is indicated by the fact that they invited him to speak at their 1966 conference. Again there is no indication that, in doing this, they were succumbing to the allure of the counter-culture. They were still very much a part of 'the establishment', so much so that some of Laing's more radical associates wondered publicly why he agreed to take part, and they retained a high level of establishment formality and etiquette at the conference. Amongst other things Mass was said at the Westminster Cathedral for members of the conference and a service was held in the chapel at Church House (Laing 1997, 120). According to his son, this kind of establishment occasion tended to bring out the rebel in Laing.

> He came to the conclusion that his twenty minutes would be best served by informing the assembled throng of the therapeutic benefits of LSD and mescaline, of the non-existence of schizophrenia, of the necessity of healing oneself before attempting to treat others, and that schizophrenia 'remains one of the greatest scandals and challenges of our time'.
>
> (Ibid.)

He was clearly *en route* to his final, irreversible passage from the establishment to the anti-establishment. NAMH representatives must have anticipated that he might make such a speech, however. His reputation went ahead of him. And there is no indication that he caused a great stir by what he said. NAMH members might not have agreed with every word he said but they were open-minded enough to want to hear his views.

NAMH had a more rocky relationship with another source of antipsychiatric criticism, however: scientology. Scientology was an object of considerable concern in the media and Parliament throughout the 1960s, resulting in a Parliamentary investigation in 1971 (Foster 1971). The cult is best known for its religious claims but it also makes strong claims regarding mental health, as is indicated by the sub-title of one of its founding texts, *Dianetics: The Modern Science of Mental Health*.[2] Moreover, in the 1970s it mounted a vehement critique of psychiatry, which it claimed was a key player in a conspiracy to control the world. For their part psychiatrists replied with criticisms of scientologists. They argued, amongst other things, that its therapeutic techniques were akin to brainwashing and caused mental breakdown amongst the vulnerable and impressionable persons it tended to attract (Wallis 1976).

This conflict between psychiatry and scientology inevitably extended to NAMH, who both identified and were identified with the psychiatric establishment at the time. When *Dianetics* was reviewed in *Mental Health* in 1952, for example, the reviewer not only complained that its ideas were 'not supported by any statistics or experimental data', a deficiency elided by use of 'Hollywood language', but also '... hope[d] that the craze for it will be short lived and that the system will soon find its way into the limbo of other extravagant creeds' (*Mental Health* 1952, XI(3), 137–8). This conflict escalated through the 1960s. The scientologists brought a number of legal cases against NAMH,[3] because of the coverage NAMH afforded scientology in *Mental Health*. NAMH were a central agency of the psychiatric establishment in the view of the scientologists and, as a consequence, were a target for scathing criticism and attack. This included demonstrations outside NAMH headquarters, including those of CAPA. Banners with the slogans 'Psychiatrists Maim and Kill' and 'Buy Your Meat from a Psychiatrist' were publicly paraded (Wallis 1976).

The antagonism peaked in 1969. In the 'eleventh hour', before an important meeting which was to involve elections to key posts within the organisation, NAMH officials noticed a recent surge in membership. Around three hundred new members had joined the organisation within a matter of months. Moreover, some amongst the three hundred had been nominated as candidates for office by others from that grouping. If a majority amongst the three hundred voted for these candidates, there was a very good chance that the latter would be elected. The new members were scientologists. NAMH had been infiltrated by its adversaries. The scientologists were attempting to take the organisation over from within. Having realised just in time, NAMH insisted on the resignation of the members, prompting a legal challenge, but the matter was ultimately settled in their favour (Wallis 1973, 1976).

## A change of MIND

The near miss with the scientologists, combined with a shortage of funds, prompted NAMH to organise a new campaign which would both replenish resources and help it to clarify its aims and policies. Some felt that the organisation had lost its direction and identity, that it was drifting. Successful infiltration by its adversaries symbolised that; the giant had been sleeping, with almost fatal consequences. Lack of funds was a sign too, however, as well as an impediment. SMOs which lack money lack the means to act, and once affluent SMOs which now lack money have evidently taken their eye off the ball.

The new campaign, the MIND campaign, ran from 1970 to 1973. And it proved to be much more than a one-off campaign. MIND became NAMH's permanent campaigning name and this name change signified a larger change of direction. Under the name MIND, NAMH were to be much more of an active political campaign group, becoming more involved in protest and the active promotion of policy change. In the years that followed they embraced a civil rights discourse, lobbied parliament fiercely and tried in various ways to change and tackle what they perceived to be the injustices of the mental health system. This was also reflected in the name (and direction) change of their journal; first, to *MIND and Mental Health*, second, to *Mind Out*, and finally to *Open Mind*. The editorial of the first issue of MIND OUT, published in 1973, conveys clearly the change in direction.

> ...MIND OUT will be dealing with subjects like controversial treatment methods, patients rights, relatives rights, legal problems posed by mentally disturbed offenders, community mental health services provided by your local authority, hospital services, public prejudice, child guidance and voluntary action to right wrongs and change attitudes.
>
> (Reproduced in *Open Mind* 50, 12–13)

Although an element of the older NAMH perspective remained (e.g. the continued concern with child guidance), this statement clearly indicated a change of direction, towards a concern with rights, wrongs and controversial treatments. Furthermore, where older concerns were retained they were often reframed. Where concern with public prejudice had once been framed in terms of the discourse of mental hygiene, with its stress upon early treatment, for example, the concern now was more related to the effects of public prejudice upon the civil rights and quality of life of those diagnosed mentally ill. The medical frame was at least rejoined, if not replaced, by a moral and political frame.

When MIND OUT became *Open Mind* in 1983, there was an effort to expand this transformation further by opening debate out to the public. *Open Mind* should, it was argued in its first issue, be more than a voice for MIND. It should facilitate debate between different viewpoints and open up its range of concerns to cover issues that had a wider public interest. Clearly, this involves some departure from the paternalism that I have identified with the early NAMH in Chapter 4. Moreover, another decisive step in this more critical direction involved the opening, in the early 1970s, of a Legal and Welfare Rights department. Larry Gostin, a civil rights lawyer from the United States, was appointed as its first legal director.

These changes dislodged MIND from its position in 'the establishment', generating tensions with both psychiatrists and the government. By the 1990s, in an interview in *Open Mind* with the president of the *Royal College of Psychiatry*, for example, MIND were able to refer in a very matter of fact fashion to the '... background of tension between MIND and the Royal College' (*Open Mind* 66, 1994, 18–19). Similarly, though the chair of the organisation in the mid 1980s was still a Lord, active in the House and able to use his position to advance MIND's aims, its changing direction was making this elite connection more uncomfortable and conflicted. In 1985, during a debate on the care of mental patients in the second chamber, for example, Lord Ennals was asked for reassurance that MIND did not support 'patient power' and 'evil' groups such as the CAPO (*Open Mind* 19, 1986, 4; on CAPO, not be confused with CAPA, see Chapter 8). Such associations, disassociations and tensions would have been unthinkable to the NAMH of the 1940s and the 1950s.

A key turning point in this shift was the publication, in 1975, of Gostin's (1975) *A Human Condition*, a two volume study which laid out a 'rights-based approach' to mental illness and criticised existing policy and practice. As a MIND retrospective, which clearly relishes in the more risqué position of the contemporary organisations, put it:

> [the study] caused an unsettling chill amongst philanthropists and professionals: prominent psychiatrists resigned from MIND's Council of Management, innuendoes were heard in government circles that MIND's funding was in jeopardy, and many believed that the beneficent traditions of MIND and psychiatry itself were being threatened.
>
> (*Open Mind* 47, 1990, 12–13)

Under the influence of Gostin and others MIND assumed a strong lobbying position. They put pressure on government and media, and mounted legal cases in both the British and European courts. In particular they called for major reforms to the 1959 Mental Health Act. The reforms came in the shape of a number of amendments to the act in 1982, followed by a new act in 1983 which effectively rewrote the legal framework for mental health services in the United Kingdom. MIND is widely credited and criticised, in equal measure, for their key role in both prompting and shaping this act (Rose 1986).

## Explaining the transformation

The episode with the scientologists was a significant trigger event in relation to NAMH's transformation. It prompted reflection and afforded an opportunity for those who wanted to bring about change. The organisation was shaken up and, like an individual who comes close to losing their life, inclined to take stock. In itself, however, it cannot explain the change in direction. NAMH might, after all, have elected to become more conservative after their 'fright'. The near success of the scientologists might have led them to seek out stronger bonds with the establishment and to take a firmer line with critics of psychiatry. The shortage of funds was more decisive. Whatever their persuasion, without money they could not function. More importantly, the shortage of money was symptomatic of a broader dynamic. The 1960s had been a period of change, particularly amongst the educated middle classes. Traditional charities appeared old fashioned and out of touch in this context, and their paternalistic stance conflicted with new ways of thinking, based in libertarian ideologies and the discourse of civil rights. This cultural drift may have permeated the thinking of NAMH officials. More importantly, however, as a shift within the educated middle classes, it affected NAMH's key constituents. NAMH relied upon the support of the middle classes. If middle class outlooks were changing, then NAMH would have to change too or die. The decline in NAMH's funds, which informed the original MIND campaign, suggests that this pressure was beginning to bite. NAMH had lost its appeal amongst its traditional constituencies and it was forced, for a second time (see Chapter 4), to reinvent itself. Demand in the political market, to borrow Zald and McCarthy's (1994) metaphor, had shifted and 'suppliers' had to shift with it.

Furthermore, as they did so they were inclined to both attract and seek to recruit more progressive types within their organisational ranks, Gostin being the obvious example of this, thus shifting the balance of power attaching to particular discourses on mental health within the organisation itself. Adherents of the civil rights discourse grew in number relative to representatives of mental hygiene and/or a more conservative position.

This pressure would have affected many charities but NAMH were particularly affected on account of the impact of both anti-psychiatry and the various scandals, critiques and civil rights campaigns that had 'plagued' psychiatry through the 1950s and 1960s. The popular image of psychiatry had never been great and one of NAMH's key self-appointed tasks during the 1940s, 1950s and 1960s had been to try and improve it, so as to enable to psychiatry to better do its job. As the public image of psychiatry and particularly its reputation amongst middle class 'conscience constituents' sank to new depths, however, NAMH risked sinking with it. Few people shared the scientologist's view of psychiatry, either within or outside of the educated middle classes, but the scientology episode indicates how easily the image of NAMH, as an apologist for traditional psychiatry, combined with its efforts to defend psychiatry against its critics, could lead to it being drawn into that criticism and conflict. Psychiatry, as a publicly funded service, was in a reasonable position to weather this storm, albeit with some adjustments, but NAMH depended upon charitable funding and thus upon its good reputation and image.

In this sense we can see how the anti-psychiatric and civil rights (e.g. NCCL) SMOs were able to exert an indirect impact upon NAMH. Both, to some degree, drew upon the same constituencies as NAMH. They were in positions of structural equivalence with it. The widespread appeal of anti-psychiatry and civil rights therefore had consequences for NAMH. It made them less attractive and popular. And this affected their donations, generating a pressure which ultimately led them to change direction. MIND did not become anti-psychiatric. That would have been a distance to great to travel in one step and, in any case, would have been unwise strategically, both because anti-psychiatry occupied that particular niche in the market, leaving little space for competitors, and because it was an extreme niche which a large and longstanding organisation would not have found conducive to long-term health. Even those who were 'mad about R.D. Laing' may have been reluctant to fund him. And many other conscience constituents, not to mention government funders, were more likely sympathetic to civil rights-based critique than to the extremes. Continued funding and thus survival required a more balanced shift. Of course there will have been more factors at work in NAMH's transformation than this; many internal to the organisation. But there is every reason to believe that the impact of anti-psychiatry, via shared conscience constituents, was strong.

## Paradigm shifts and resource flows

In Chapters 4 and 5 I referred to a paradigm shift in the field of psychiatric contention which, I argued, anti-psychiatry had some part in bringing about. What I am discussing now is both an effect and a mechanism of that shift. When the ground of dominant sentiments and discourse shifts SMOs dependent upon wider sentiment pools for their survival have a very strong incentive to shift with them, whatever they might think about the changes. This is an effect of the shift; a shift, in this case, which is partly attributable to anti-psychiatric SMOs but also to the wider current of the 1960s, to which it belonged.

NAMH's radical change of/into MIND wasn't only an effect of the shift, however, it was a major mechanism in the advancement and completion of that shift. MIND was a big organisation with a lot of weight to throw behind its campaigns. It was a major player. When MIND changed direction, therefore, the balance of power and opinion in the field shifted. In addition, MIND was in possession of considerable resources (money, networks, offices, channels of communication etc.) which it made available to other, smaller SMOs. When it became more radical, therefore, resource flows for more conservative projects dried up, simultaneously becoming available to more progressive and critical projects. Such a shift in resource flows, as Zald and McCarthy (1994) suggest, can be a major stimulus for the development of new projects and SMOs. In accordance with my value-added model, it represents an important shift in conditions of structural conduciveness. And the evidence, some of which we see in Chapter 8, suggests that the transformation of NAMH had just this effect. A number of the SMOs that I discuss in Chapter 8 received grants from MIND; many operated from MIND premises; many self-publicised through *Open Mind*; and many came together by way of MIND's events and its wider network. As noted in Chapter 4, MIND was like a vast ganglia running through the mental health field, connecting interested parties at the local, regional, national and international levels. The more receptive the organisation became to critical currents of thought, the more available these networks became to the radically inclined. They became effective mobilising structures. NAMH's transformation into MIND was a major factor inducing paradigm shift in the field of contention because it involved a major transformation of resource flows within the field.

Related to this, MIND's strong network of local and regional offices (see Chapter 4), combined with its image as progressive, critical and civil rights oriented but also respectable and safe, made it an important recruitment filter for the field. Most of the more critical activists I spoke to had some involvement in MIND and many had started their activist careers with it. There were different reasons for this, not least of which was its resource base, but in some cases it was also noted that MIND was a less intimidating point of contact than some of the more radical groups in play within the field. They were an easier channel of involvement for agents who were finding their feet in the world of mental health politics.

Not everybody was happy with the changes in psycho-politics, however. The emphasis upon 'patients' rights' and related criticisms of psychiatric labels and power were creating their own problems in the views of some. This really came to a head in the 1980s, as we see in Chapter 9. The first seeds of this movement were sown in the 1970s, however, with the birth of the *National Schizophrenia Fellowship* (NSF).

## Relative reactions

The NSF was founded in 1972. The origins of its formation lie in an anonymous letter written to *The Times* in 1970 by the group's founder, John Pringle. Pringle's son was a diagnosed schizophrenic. It had taken two years for this diagnosis to be arrived at, however. In the first instance, this was because of the manner in which the relevant authorities at his university responded to his behaviour, which became erratic and dissociated. The college failed to identify what Pringle himself identified as mental illness. To them it was simply unsuitable behaviour. Second, psychiatrists and welfare workers proved little better. According to Pringle's analysis this was due, in large part, to an unwillingness of psychiatrists to apply a 'dreaded label'. He claimed to understand this reluctance, even if he was irritated by the 'weary platitudes' of those psychiatrists and welfare workers who urged him to be patient. The cost, however, was a considerable delay in any help being offered to his son. Another part of the problem in Pringle's view, moreover, was the level of general disorganisation and lack of communication within the health and welfare services. And this continued after the diagnosis had been made. Indeed, Pringle noted the general lack of organisation and consequent lack of care for schizophrenics, particularly those who were 'well enough' to live in the community but still considerably disabled by their illness. Compassion for the patient was a key theme in the letter but more central still was the perspective of those who live with and care for him or her. Anticipating the key campaigning issue of the NSF, Pringle noted that mental hospitals were being closed at a far greater rate than alternative provisions were being put into place, leaving the immediate circle of the patient, particularly the family, to pick up the shortfall. Even when drugs have dampened the worst symptoms of the illness, he argued, this is a considerable burden, not least because the behaviour and experience of the schizophrenic defies the standard mechanisms of interpersonal interaction and understanding. This experience, Pringle added, had prompted him to discover if other families were in a similar situation. He found that they were.

Pringle's letter generated many responses from families around the United Kingdom who were also in a similar situation and it was this response and the connections between similarly situated individuals and families that it generated which both prompted and facilitated the formation of the NSF as a national organisation. Initially the organisation consisted of only a small number of people. By the late 1980s, however, it had grown into a major organisation with over 6000 members, 150 local support groups and more than 300 staff (undated NSF flyer). Moreover, they were keen to enlist the support of sympathetic and influential professionals, who shared their concern about the often neglected social dynamics and consequences of both mental illness and its treatment.

The NSF portrayed itself as a progressive organisation and in many respects bore the hallmarks one might expect of such an organisation. It was critical of government, particularly in relation to the gap between hospital closure and provision of new community services. And it involved patients in its activities, arguably in greater numbers than any other mental health SMO at the time. It was a controversial organisation, however, branded as reactionary by many involved in MIND and related groups, and attacked on these grounds. From the critics' point of view, NSF sided with those who often sought to have their 'inconvenient' relatives dealt with, those who some anti-psychiatric theories suggested were responsible for the patient's distress in the first place (the family). And they sought to promote the labels and diagnostic categories that self-styled 'radicals' were equally keen to challenge. In effect, the NSF were calling for a more robust use of psychiatric labels and interventions, quicker diagnoses and treatment with more drugs and less equivocation, whilst MIND were challenging labels and interventions. The NSF believed that schizophrenia was real and that the problems surrounding it stemmed from the fact that too few people were aware of this. They believed that psychiatric paternalism was both justified and necessary because, by definition, schizophrenics were not in control of their own lives and, in some cases, failed to recognise that they were ill and needed help. Many in MIND, by contrast, were of the view that schizophrenia was a convenient label which, in itself, often was 'the problem', and sought to challenge psychiatric paternalism on civil rights and other political grounds.

The NSF were not acting in ignorance of the views of MIND or the anti-psychiatrists, however. Indeed, they believed these groups and their discourses to be 'part of the problem' (the reverse was also true). Though their main campaign efforts were devoted to a critique of failures in community care, they were also critical of what they perceived to be misguided liberalism, which hampered effective interventions, legitimated the closure of much needed mental hospitals and compounded public ignorance regarding mental illness. The NSF were, in some part, a backlash against anti-psychiatric and civil libertarian currents in psychiatry. They were a 'counter-movement'. Needless to say, the archive records a variety of tussles around these issues, at least in the form of exchanges in mental health journals.

I will return to these conflicts. First, however, I want to reflect, as I have for the other groups but more briefly,[4] upon the conditions which gave rise to the formation of this SMO. The policy shift from hospital to community care and towards greater outpatient and day patient facilities, called for in 1959 (Chapter 3), was beginning to put a strain on the families of the mentally ill in the 1970s, and this was exacerbated by the fact that the main critical voices in the public sphere (anti-psychiatry and the civil rights lobby) were calling for a further reduction of psychiatric intervention, and were sometimes laying the blame for mental health problems on the family. Families felt desperate and angry. Structurally there was nothing to prevent them from speaking out about this, no lack of political opportunities, except perhaps the stigmatisation that attached to the mentally ill and to their families, an obstacle which, paradoxically, the liberals were going some way to dismantling. Group formation requires a trigger, however. And it requires channels of communication and mobilising structures. The *Times* article provided both. It sparked like-minded people into action, simultaneously linking them via their common link to Pringle. By writing his article Pringle became the hub of a network of like-minded critics. A further SMO had entered the field of psychiatric contention.

## Conclusion

In this chapter I have examined a number of significant developments in the field of psychiatric contention from the early 1970s: the transformation of NAMH into MIND and the formation, respectively, of PNP and the NSF. In each case I have offered both a narrative, processual account of events and a more abstract analytical dissection based upon my concept of fields and my value-added model. I will return to these SMOs later in the study. What I have also tried to begin to show in this chapter, however, is the way in which the field of contention operates as a field. None of the SMOs discussed in this chapter existed in isolation. PNP emerged, to some degree, out of the discourse and networks of anti-psychiatry and its SMOs: the PA and IPS. NAMH became MIND, in part, because civil rights and anti-psychiatric SMOs had changed the climate of mental health campaigning and, importantly, in doing so had contributed a transformation of the constituency NAMH relied upon for funds. It was structurally equivalent to anti-psychiatric and civil rights SMOs and therefore inevitably affected by their activities. And NSF, as the chief SMO in an emerging counter-movement, defined itself in opposition to the trends and currents represented by PNP, the PA, IPS and MIND. As a representative of a counter-movement, its very identity was dependent upon those movements and SMOs which it opposed. Moreover, these groups and movements were not the only players in the field during the 1970s, as we will see in Chapter 7.

# 7   A union of mental patients

The formation of the NSF and the transformation of NAMH into MIND, or at least the shape that both NSF and MIND assumed in their early years, whilst not reducible to the field effects generated by anti-psychiatry were certainly influenced, in different ways, by them. We cannot fully understand either SMO without taking account of anti-psychiatry and their relationship to it. In this chapter I focus on another development in the 1970s which was shaped by the anti-psychiatry effect, though again without being reducible to it, and another SMO which came into conflict with both MIND and the NSF, as well as the anti-psychiatrists. The focus of the chapter is the birth of the *Mental Patients' Union* (MPU).

The MPU is important because, although it is not the first example of protest activity by psychiatric patients in the history of the mental health services (see Chapter 3), it is the first link in an unbroken chain of 'patient' activism which leads through to the present day. The MPU were pre-dated slightly by a *Scottish Union of Mental Patients* (SUMP), who formed in 1971, but this group folded relatively quickly and although its founder did later link up with some MPU members there is no direct line of influence from SUMP to the MPU, as there is from the MPU to many of the groups still active today. In this respect the birth of MPU was the birth of the modern survivor movement.

## Origins and philosophy

The MPU emerged out of a successful strike at the Paddington Day Hospital (PDH), a democratic therapeutic community in London, in 1971. The strike was a response to a proposal by the local hospital group that the PDH should be closed and replaced by a more conventional outpatients unit, employing the mainstream treatments (i.e. ECT and drugs) that its current therapeutic team had rejected. The Day Hospital, which formed part of a larger institute involving both child guidance and adult outpatient units, had been established in 1962. Its original purpose was to help patients who had been discharged from a mental hospital to readjust to life on the outside but its staff, like many of their contemporaries, had been strongly influenced by the intellectual and political currents of the 1960s, and these currents had drawn it away from its original anchor point. Eventually, after the strike and partly as a consequence of it, this led to the day hospital becoming radically experimental. As in PA houses, every attempt was made to dissolve formal roles and hierarchies, instituting a form of psychotherapeutic governance that was, on the surface, radically democratic. Unlike PA houses, however, where psychoanalytic interpretation was regarded with much the same disdain as conventional psychiatry, as a clumsy and dogmatic theoretical reduction of lived experience, all aspects of organisation and activity in the Day Hospital were subject to psychoanalytic interpretation. This situation led to a second revolt at the unit, this time of patients against their psychoanalytic carers (Baron 1987). At the time of the strike, however, the hospital, which was occasionally visited by David Cooper, had not reached this extreme. An emphasis on socio-therapy, which had emerged in the mid sixties, was gradually being replaced with a more psychotherapeutic approach. Existential psychoanalysis, akin to and informed by the pioneering work of Laing, Cooper and Esterson, was being replaced by a more intra-psychic variant of (Kleinian) psychoanalysis. And many of the formal organisational distinctions of standard NHS treatment centres had been either replaced or 'democratised'. But what many patients later regarded as a tyrannical psychoanalytic regime had not yet been put in place. The Day Hospital was akin to Laing's *Rumpus Room*, *Villa 21*, even perhaps *Kingsley Hall*, and its staff, and some patients, had been directly influenced by these experiments.

The strike at the hospital, as noted, was prompted by the threatened closure of the unit. Staff mobilised. They secured the support of 22 MPs, who signed a petition, and 80 GPs, who called for the hospital to remain open. More noticeable than this, however, was the involvement of patients. They, like the staff, had much to lose by the closure of the hospital. They were faced with the prospect of a return to mainstream psychiatry, with its ECT machines and chemical side effects, not to mention an uprooting of what had become their community. But unlike the staff they had little to lose by taking part in the protest.

An orthodox psychoanalytic interpretation of the patients' fear and anger at the proposed closure would have reduced it to the intrapsychic and unconscious sphere, and to the personal history of the patient. Perhaps they had felt rejected and let down before? Perhaps their anger at the hospital board was really anger at a parental figure, a transference or projection? This is how complaints about the PDH itself were treated by its staff later in the history of the unit. The more socially and existentially engaged ideas current in the unit at the time lent themselves to an externally focused interpretation and framing, however, which in turn prompted direct action. As one of the workers, who was involved both in the strike and setting up the MPU, notes:

> When the group were informed in October 1971 of the decision to close the unit, it became part of the treatment to assess their own power in relation to this new external situation. They saw that the regional

board was relying upon their passive acceptance of the decision, and decided to refuse to be in collusion with this expectation. They issued a statement outlining their preference for psychotherapy.

(Durkin 1972, 13–15)

In this context, psychotherapy effectively functioned as political agitation. It framed emotional responses to the proposed closure in such a way as to politicise them, locating 'the problem' outside of the psychical and familiar realm, where other psychotherapies might have been inclined to locate it, in the politico-economic domain of the health authority bureaucracy. Anxious, upset and angry patients were encouraged to recognise their feelings as legitimate moral sentiments and to act upon these sentiments by way of protest. They were encouraged to overcome the feelings of power-lessness that overwhelmed some by realising, in both senses of the word, the options for resistance that were open to them. This use of psychotherapy and the framing apparatus deployed went beyond Laing and even Cooper but the influence of both is evident. They sought to bring questions of 'power' and 'collusion' – both terms are used in the above quotation – into therapy and analysis, and also to locate 'inner' problems in the 'outer' realm. The strike at the PDH, and the agitation which preceded it, set out to do this too, but in a very practical and directly political way. And polit-ically it worked. Patients were mobilised and the strike was a success. The unit was kept open. More importantly for our purposes, however, the strike provided the impetus for a decision to form a more permanent union of mental patients: the MPU.

Although a number of patients had been recruited in the strike, only one, the now legendary Eric Irwin, was involved in the initial planning commit-tee for the MPU, alongside three mental health professionals. Two other patients from outside of the Day Hospital were soon recruited via personal contacts, however, one of whom had attended anti-psychiatry meetings with David Cooper, and the core of six began planning their first meeting and writing a manifesto. This manifesto, formally titled 'The Need for a Mental Patient's Union: Some Proposals', like Irwin, has passed into move-ment legend, but under a different name: 'the Fish Manifesto'. The fish reference relates to the picture of a fish struggling on the end of a line which formed the front page of the manifesto. Under the picture, framing its meaning, was a quotation from the progressive US psychiatrist, Karl Mennenger.

An individual having unusual difficulties in coping with his environ-ment struggles and kicks up the dust, as it were. I have used the figure of a fish caught on a hook; his gyrations must look peculiar to other fish that don't understand the circumstances; but his splashes are not his affliction, they are his effort to get rid of his affliction and as every fisherman knows these efforts may succeed.

The philosophy expressed here is identical to a key theme of Laingian anti-psychiatry. Mental distress is portrayed as a purposive attempt to make sense of and cope with difficult circumstances. The opening paragraph of the manifesto marks out the distance between the proposed MPU and anti-psychiatry, however, criticising the latter on the grounds that its inner circle was exclusively composed of mental health professionals, with no patient involvement.

> In the past few years a number of groups have sprung up in opposition to the reactionary institutions of the mental hospital and psychiatry. Ignoring patient involvement, the impetus of these groups' radical alternative however, have become little more than intellectual discussion points and shop-talk for students and professionals. PATIENTS it would seem, are seen as incapable of playing any part in fighting for such alternatives.
>
> Almost colluding with the myth that mental patients are 'inadequate', these groups have dismissed completely the fact that patients, of whom most are working class, together with hospital workers and nurses, are the only agents of revolutionary change inside the mental hospital.
>
> (*Mental Patients' Union* 1972, opening paragraphs
> (pages not numbered))

Furthermore, the entire manifesto is strongly framed in Marxist terms. This framing resonates with Cooper but not Laing, who was never a Marxist. Throughout the manifesto, the struggle of mental patients is identified as part of a wider class struggle, with mental distress being accounted for in Marxist terms: that is, alienated labour, domestic slavery and unemployment. Psychiatry, the document claims, is 'one of the most subtle methods of repression in advanced capitalist society' (ibid.). And mental patients should form together in a union to oppose it, standing alongside other radical groups who were voicing their protest at the time: 'Trade Unions, Claimants' Unions, Women's Liberation, Black Panther Groups, Prisoner's Rights' (ibid.).

The prospect of learning from and uniting with these other groups was not unrealistic. Most of the members of the original planning group had previous and current involvement with these and other groups, as one explained to me: '[name] and I were involved for a while in the Claimants' Union. I'd also been involved in PROP [a prisoners' rights organisation]. [different name] was in what's now the Socialist Workers Party (SWP)' (Interview 2, patient and MPU activist).

Indeed, this interviewee suggested that two of the founder members of the MPU were members of the organisation which was to become the SWP; that is, the International Socialists (IS). In addition, one of the founders, Liz Durkin, had published a pamphlet with the Young Fabians on *Hostels for the Mentally Disordered* (Durkin 1971). The presence of IS members within the MPU is significant because, like many Trotskyist organisations, the IS had a tendency towards agitation, in Blumer's (1969) sense (see Chapter 2); that is, towards mobilising populations involved in a conflict by framing their conflict, organising them and equipping them for protest, even to the point, on some occasions, of forming its own 'front' SMO to engage in these conflicts. In addition, it should come as no surprise that the *Fish Manifesto* was couched in strongly Marxist language, given that two out of its original four members were IS members.

I do not mean to suggest that the MPU was a front for the IS. It was not. Furthermore, much of the MPU's early profile could be accounted for in other terms. Britain in the 1970s, like other European and North American countries, was in the latter stages of a wave of contention and Marxism and the language and tactics of workers' struggles (e.g. 'unions' and 'strikes') had become a central discourse and 'master frame' in radical circles. A variety of players in non-labour-based struggles had appropriated them. It wasn't just mental patients who formed a *'union'* and *'went on strike'* at this time. As the above quotation reminds us, benefits claimants formed a union too, and housing tenants went on strike. In addition, as the concept of waves of contention suggests (see Chapter 2), this was a time when conflict was proliferating across a range of *prima facie* unconnected domains, both as agents in these domains found inspiration from the evidence of other struggles around them and sought to keep up, and as the 'political entrepreneurs' involved in these other struggles, finding themselves in increasingly crowded 'markets', sought to diversify, carving out new niche markets of struggle. The culture of politicisation and struggle was spreading rapidly and the agency of the IS was only one factor in this spread. Nevertheless, the presence of IS at the heart of the MPU cannot have been without significance and effect.

The opposition of the original fish activists to anti-psychiatry, to return briefly to that, is important. The MPU, as a new group, was seeking out a niche within the field of psychiatric contention and seeking to depose anti-psychiatry from its dominant position therein. It was in a 'structurally equivalent', if less influential position to the anti-psychiatric SMOs within the field. It appealed to the same pool of adherents/constituents and opposed the same practices and elites. This generated a strategic incentive for the MPU to mark out its difference from and superiority to the anti-psychiatrists. If it wasn't different to anti-psychiatry and didn't believe that aspects of anti-psychiatry were problematic then why generate a different group? In spite of their criticism, however, early MPU activists continued to reference anti-psychiatric writing positively in their own writing, thereby acknowledging the influence of the anti-psychiatrists upon them. Indeed, many early MPU publications contain 'reading lists' comprising books and articles which central figures in the MPU wished to recommend to their less-informed readers, and the texts of Laing, Cooper, Esterson,

Berke, Schatzman, as well as Goffman, Szasz, Scheff and others, all figure prominently. This reveals the rather more complex and dialectical nature of the relation of the MPU's discourse to that of anti-psychiatry. The MPU's discourse had emerged out of a dialogue with that of anti-psychiatry, sparked by the explosive impact and influence of the latter. As such the former incorporated aspects of the latter whilst simultaneously rejecting, revising and reframing other aspects. The MPU were similar to PNP in this respect. The discourses of both were, on one level, replies or responses to anti-psychiatry which absorbed much of it even as they marked out their difference from it. In the case of the MPU, however, the marked-out difference was greater.

The anti-psychiatrists were not the only targets of early MPU critique. MIND too were now pretenders to the crown of psychiatric criticism and they too came under criticism from the MPU. One particular bone of contention was the use of ECT, particularly in instances where that use was against the patient's wishes. MIND, at this point in time, still condoned the practice but MPU activists were very critical. A number of exchanges on this issue can be found in their respective journals. At a more general level, however, in an article first published in 1975,[1] MPU founder, Eric Irwin, and co-author Mary Hutchins, mounted a scathing critique of MIND's 'liberalism'. MIND's analysis, they argued, 'lacks any rigorous class critique of society', and

> MIND's optimistic liberalism, therefore, can at best lead to no more than a passive reinforcement of traditional psychiatric norms. It can only serve to perpetuate, in failing to truly expose psychiatry, the ideology of the existing ruling class and its oppression. MIND's patching-up community approach (which community is puzzling) thus appears to be an apologia for present government structure or a public relations job for 'charitable' housing trusts.
>
> (Irwin and Hutchins 1975)

The MPU were staking out the radical ground for themselves, positioning themselves relative to other groups in a structurally equivalent position and competing for symbolic dominance. They were the most radical players in the game and the others, the liberals, missed the point.

MIND, for their part, had been supportive of the strike of the PDH and organised a press conference in an effort to help. They had not yet arrived at the idea of 'patient power', however. Patient members of the PDH action group were not initially invited to the press conference and, when admitted, found themselves organised out of the proceedings. 'The group queried this and finally, though it was seen as a 'novel idea', they were invited. However the conference was structured and hierarchical and the patients were effectively unable to participate' (Durkin 1972: 13–15).

## Back to the fish manifesto

*The Fish Manifesto* outlines four areas where an MPU could become active. First, they could 'propagandise', exposing the injustices of the system and informing patients of the 'minimal' rights they enjoyed at the time. Second, they could establish a 'Charter of Rights', covering such rights as the '... the right to a second opinion...to refuse treatment...to retain [one's own] clothing in hospital...' and 'to effective appeal machinery'. Third, they could fight and campaign on a number of issues, including the 'abolition of compulsory admissions and treatment, of irreversible treatments and the use of isolation rooms for "disruptive" patients', and of the censorship and surveillance of phone calls and letters. The end goal, in this respect, was 'the abolition of mental hospitals and the institution of repressive and manipulative psychiatry.' Finally, they could set up alternatives to psychiatry, in the form of drop-in and live-in centres. All of this, the manifesto insisted, should be under the control of patients.

> The Union would be organised and controlled only by mental patients and ex-patients. The Union membership and voting rights would be limited to patients alone. The union must be run democratically with an effective working group elected and subject to the right of recall. Outside help would be more than welcome, but would only carry associate membership with no voting rights.
>
> (MPU 1971)

The demands are paradoxical on at least two counts. First, they are surprisingly liberal and pragmatic, given the revolutionary language elsewhere evident in the manifesto. The focus on rights, for example, belongs to liberal rather than Marxist discourse, and the rights called for generally accord with a liberal conception of 'the rights of man' (e.g. to privacy, autonomy etc.). MPU discourse comprised a Marxist and anti-psychiatric analysis of the situation of mental patients with liberal and anti-psychiatric moral claims-making. Second, the emphasis on the privilege to be accorded to patients sits somewhat oddly with the fact that 3 out of the 6 members on the organising committee, and 3 out of the 4 members of that committee at its inception, were mental health workers rather than patients. This is a paradox which occurs time and again in relation to the patient/survivor movement. I will return to it.

When the manifesto was written it was distributed in advance of the proposed foundational meeting of the Union: '... we put a lot of effort into distributing it. I think it had quite an effect. ... it went into a lot of hospitals, psychiatric units' (Interview 2).

These distribution efforts involved blind mails shots but also drew upon the vast informal network that psychiatric practices produce as a 'side effect'. As patients and mental health workers move through different hospital units relationships form which connect individuals, institutions and their populations. At the individual level, each patient has a personal network of fellow patients and 'friendly' workers whom they have met in the course of their psychiatric career. And as contacts disperse to new and different units, their personal network functions to link their new institutions and the relevant others in those institutions. By means of such a network the *Fish Manifesto* and the idea of a mental patients union were able to spread, along with the details of the MPU's inaugural meeting: 21st March 1973 at the PDH.

However, whatever the effects of the manifesto, mail shot and informal network, events overtook the organising committee. The media became interested in them, reporting upon their proposed formation, coining numerous labels to describe them, including 'mad lib', and thereby generating a considerable degree of publicity. Node-to-node diffusion received a boost from the broadcast networks (in both senses of the term[2]) of the mass media. Particularly significant, in the view of the organising committee, was an interview on Radio Four's *Today* programme, the day before the inaugural meeting. The circumstances of the interview are revealing. Although the producers of the programme were interested in the idea of a union of mental patients and wanted to interview a representative of the union, they did not want to interview a mental patient. They wanted to interview one of the professionals involved. The organising committee refused, arguing that it had to be one of the patients. After a long negotiation, which ran through the night, the producers of the programme agreed. The organising committee elected one of their patient members to be interviewed.

The increased diffusion and excitement generated by media coverage led to significant 'amplification' of the event reported. Attendance at the meeting far exceeded expectations and room capacity: '... we thought that we would get from six to eight or twenty and we got over, I forget what the number was, I guess 150. It was a really crowded meeting' (Interview 2, patient and MPU member).

*Radio 4* had inadvertently connected a small cell of activists with a section of their potential constituency. The idea of a mental patients union became mobile, moving 'through the wires' and initially positioning the organising committee at the hub of an enormous network 'wheel' (see Figure 7.1). The wheel crashed inwards almost immediately, however, as its 'nodes', by way of the first meeting, came into contact. Relations of mutual acquaintance forged at the first meeting reshaped the network structure as a dense weave of would-be activists. Geographically dispersed and isolated (from one another) individuals had become a group (Figure 7.1).

The MPU was born, with a large constituency, and it continued to grow. Cells emerged elsewhere in London and throughout the United Kingdom, including Manchester, Leeds, Oxford and Surrey. Figures indicating this growth are difficult to assess, not least because, as one MPU interviewee informed me, his colleague, who produced the official figures, had a tendency

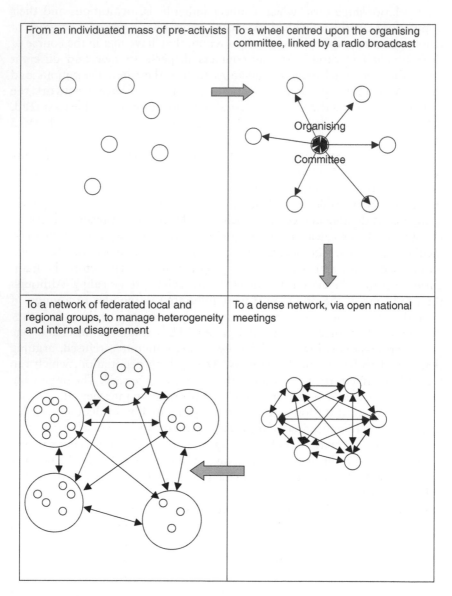

*Figure 7.1* The evolving network structure of the MPU.

to inflate them somewhat for purposes of self-presentation. Using these figures the MPU membership rose to between 500 and 600 in a relatively short period. A more reliable measure, based upon the members cards that were used for mailing, however, suggest a membership of 314 in March 1974, rising to between 375 and 400 by July 1974, before dropping to 269 in

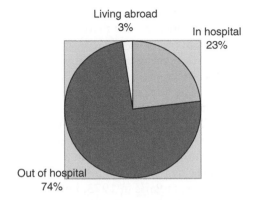

Living abroad
3%

In hospital
23%

Out of hospital
74%

*Figure 7.2* MPU membership in March 1974 (n = 314).

January of 1975 (the archive stops at this point). One new member, interestingly, was David Cooper, who also brought a small circle of his peers with him. Cooper had been out of the country at the time the MPU formed but returned shortly afterwards. As a recovering alcoholic, he registered as a full (i.e. 'patient') member. Membership dues, in the first year, were five pence per month for patients and ten pence for ex-patients, though advertising stressed that waivers were possible. Associate members, that is, members who had never been diagnosed as mentally ill, paid two pounds per year.

A membership breakdown for March 1974 suggests that the largest proportion of members, by a considerable margin, were living outside of hospital (see Figure 7.2). This skew is odd from one point of view. Hospitalised patients are in the closest proximity of all patients to the conditions that the MPU were challenging, so we might expect them to be most involved. There are better reasons to explain the opposite, actual pattern, however. First, patients in hospital may be less capable of partaking in collective action, either as a consequence of the mental distress for which they are being treated, given that one would expect patients to be hospitalised at those times when they are most distressed, or as one amongst the many side effects of that treatment, given that incapacitating treatment regimes are more likely in the hospital context for a mix of good and bad reasons.[3] Second, however, there is good evidence that MPU activism was resisted by some professionals within the hospital context, in a manner that was not possible outside of it. Specifically there is evidence that posters advertising meetings were ripped from walls and that some patients who showed an interest were subject to intimidation and/or had their medication increased. To cite a particular case, Sedgwick reports that: 'A serious battle had to be waged by the MPU branch at Hackney Hospital to secure permission for its meetings there; most hospitals and staff find the idea of independent and collective patient action threatening to their own status' (Sedgwick 1982, 228). In this particular case a group of MPU activists from outside of Hackney visited the hospital, demanding that meetings be allowed to go ahead and threatening to generate publicity if they were not. Hospital staff conceded but there were other less successful instances and we do not know about cases where intimidation was sufficiently successful as to ensure its own invisibility. Thus it seems equally likely that hospitalised patients were less well represented in the MPU because they were subject to greater control. The hospital was less 'structurally conducive' to protest and group formation (see Chapter 2).

Alongside national proliferation, the MPU became networked with various groups overseas, specifically in France, Germany, Holland, Spain, Canada and the United States. The only joint action I have been able to discover in relationship to this network involved six members of the MPU meeting up with French, Spanish and German groups, in Paris in 1973, both for a conference and to mount a joint protest at the German embassy against the treatment of political prisoners in Germany. The psychiatric link in this protest came from the fact that the German group, *Sozialistisches Patienten Kollectiv* (SPK), had been linked by the German authorities to the *Red Army Faction*. Their occupation of their hospital in Heidelberg had been subject to a SWAT-type raid on the grounds that they were believed to be storing guns and bomb-making equipment (Spandler 1992). Some had been arrested and others had fled the country. Those who were still free therefore wished to protest in the interests of those who were incarcerated. This international network also met the following year in Amsterdam, this time assumedly with Dutch groups too, but to my knowledge there were no further joint actions. The primary function of the network was to transmit ideas and offer mutual (verbal) support.

The growth of the MPU meant an increase in its resources. Newly formed links between people were, in themselves, a form of social capital. And each of the nodes in those links, the new cells/members brought their own personal resources with them. Each individual joining a cell had skills, material and cultural goods, social positions and wider connections that could be pooled and mobilised in the context of struggle. This surge in resources enabled the MPU, relatively early its history, to extend the 'shopstewardly' representation (Sedgwick 1982, 228) it sought to offer its members by engaging a solicitor and taking up a number of legal battles. As one MPU newsletter from 1973 explained:

THE UNION HAS A SOLICITOR willing to give free advice and to act for us. We are presently fighting the case of a girl incarcerated by her mother's authority in a mental hospital...against her will...coerced 'voluntarily'. She is denied visitors and correspondence. We have the support of her teachers who are upset by this since it is interrupting her schooling. She is coming up to her A-Levels. More news in the next newsletter. WRITE TO THIS OFFICE IF YOU NEED LEGAL HELP. (emphasis in original)

In addition to legal representation, the MPU appears to have focused its energies on two key domains of activity. First, it produced a relatively large number of publications. In addition to manifestos and regular newsletters, a number of cells were active in the production of pamphlets addressing issues of concern for psychiatric patients. One of the most important examples of this was a *Directory of Psychiatric Drugs* which discussed the various drugs prescribed by psychiatrists and their effects. Such publications had the obvious effect of arming patients with information that would be of use both in personal decisions about treatment and in any conflicts over treatment they may become involved in with psychiatrists. Furthermore, they generated a critical public within the mental health field, intersecting with that produced by Laing *et al.* and serving to keep psychiatry in question. Second, some MPU cells set up squats which became both their headquarters and 'crash houses'. Like the publications, which were facilitated by the involvement of MPU members in underground publishing networks, the use of crash house squats involved the mobilisation of a range of social connections and practical skills located within the alternative and countercultural scene of the time. In the case of the first London-based house, for example, the key player was Robin Farquharson, who, along with Michael Barnett of PNP and Leon Redler of the PA, via the *Situationist Housing Association*, had 'arranged' a house for PNP too. Furthermore, one 'protohacker' within the MPU devised a way of wiring up a telephone in one of the squats without going through the official channels, so as to provide a free telephone service. MPU members may have been relatively poor in terms of the conventional goods of UK society, the goods that sociologists often take as indicators of wealth and power, but they were rich in certain 'counter-cultural goods', not least of which were skills in subverting and working 'the system' for one's own benefit and connectedness to the network of the counter-culture, with the further skills and resources that could be mobilised therein. This is significant because it illustrates, whilst modifying a basic point emphasised in much social movement literature; namely, that mobilisation presupposes social capital and resources. The modification occurs because we can see that and how alternative and underground cultures generate a range of their own resources which have no obvious place in 'straight society'.

However involvement in alternative society also shaped the practices of the MPU in somewhat surreal ways too. A resident in a squat where one local branch held their meetings, for example, preferred to lie in her bed during meetings, in the room above the meeting room. She had smashed a hole through the ceiling/floor which allowed her to make impromptu contributions to the meetings: 'and you get her voice coming down at a crucial point in the meeting from the hole above' (Interview 2). More problematically, beyond the surrealism, radical practices generated problems which were frustrating for some. The radical democracy and openness of the group meant that everything became open to debate and collective decision, including such trivial matters as 'who would buy the loo rolls' (Interview 2). Moreover, the liberal ethos was found to have only weak defences against the illiberal currents that sometimes flowed into the union as it expanded and recruited from outside radical circles.

> ...three people came from [name], one of whom was a racist, and whoever was trying to keep that meeting together was having to avoid getting racism written into the Mental Patient Union because [he said that] one of the problems with mental hospitals was that there were too many black nurses. I mean this guy was having a field day, y' know,...In theory there was nothing to stop that being written down and that being our policy. It would have been turned over at the next meeting but...
>
> (Interview 2, patient and MPU activist)

Though extreme and specific, this case also illustrates a wider problem that beset the MPU as it grew. Though growth generated resources it also multiplied the range of viewpoints within the group to an unsustainable point. Where the planning committee for the group had shared a similar trajectory of political involvement and had arrived at a similar outlook, new members approached the issue of patient politics from very different positions and trajectories. Thus, at the formative meeting of the national MPU, following a debate and vote, *The Fish Manifesto* was rejected and it was decided that a new 'Declaration of Intent'should be drawn up. The substantive content of the new *Declaration of Intent* was quite similar to the *Fish Manifesto*. However, it is interesting that the Marxist terminology, which is very evident in the first document, was removed in the second, and with it the Marxist framing of the MPU's agenda. Although the second document still cites 'housing, unemployment and social inequalities' as significant factors in the generation of mental health problems, proclaims society to be 'sick and defective' and deems psychiatry 'repressive and manipulative', earlier references to class, capitalism, alienation etc. have been removed. Moreover, a former member of the organisation informed me that anti-psychiatry and particularly Marxism, along with issues concerning the direction and *de facto* leadership of the group, became objects of conflict and argument within it (Interview 2). The ideologies and practices of the foundational MPU cell were alien to many of the later cells that formed around it, and alienating. Newcomers, from outside of the alternative society, did not take for granted all that it took for granted and they took for granted much that it sought to question. There was a clash of cultures.

The tensions and disagreements were such that, following a second annual general meeting (AGM) in Manchester in March 1974, it was decided that the MPU should become a loose federation of autonomous local groups rather than a centralised organisation. These local groups would be connected by way of a regular newsletter, AGM and conferences, but they would be free to set their own agendas regarding ideology, tactics and activities. The mechanistic solidarity of the organising committee, based upon similarity of beliefs and approaches, gave way, if not to organic solidarity, then, at least to a liberal arrangement where some common ground was shared and local groups 'agreed to disagree' about everything else. Mechanisms of collective-identity building were not completely ejected, however. In particular, the MPU developed a very distinctive and evocative symbol, 'human head on a spider's web', which was widely used. The symbol, whose merits were debated relative to a reworking of the fish motif over the course of a number of meetings, was intended to capture the sense of an individual caught up in a web of psychiatry and social control, and was intended to look aggressive or confrontational.

The point at which the MPU federalised also provided an occasion for further defections and spin offs, one of which enjoyed a higher profile in the later history of the patients' movement than the MPU itself. I discuss this splinter group in Chapter 8. Suffice it to say for now that most MPU cells had died out by the mid-1970s, along with the formal network channels connecting them.

## Accounting for the MPU

The emergence of the MPU, outlined in narrative form earlier, can be explained in a more abstract and analytic form by way of my value-added model.

*(i) Strain*   The strains to which the members of the MPU were reacting are fairly evident from the documents they published. At a very basic level most of the patient constituency involved had been subject to psychiatric interventions which they had experienced as unpleasant, unnecessary, humiliating and, given their often compulsory nature, oppressive. They felt that psychiatrists and other mental health workers intervened into and sought to control their lives. Moreover, they felt that the labels that were imposed upon them by mental health professionals were stigmatising and misrepresented the nature of their distress. They were not ill, in their own view, they were attempting to cope with difficult circumstances. The problem did not lie with them, as individuals, but rather with the environment in which they found themselves and which made their lives difficult.

As noted in Chapter 2, strain is always relative to expectations. It arises when conditions breach expectations and is therefore as likely to be the result of a change of expectations as of external circumstances. As noted in Chapter 3, there had been important waves of reform in mental health services in both the 1930s and the late 1950s. It would be difficult to conclude, therefore, that strains were greater in the 1970s because objective conditions within psychiatry were worsening. They weren't. However, the fact of reform itself does indicate that expectations might have been rising, and perhaps at a faster pace than conditions on the ground. We need to understand the strain expressed in the claims of the MPU against this background. The patients of the 1970s were one of the first generations to have grown up with the 'enlightened' view of psychiatry that emerged between the 1930s and the 1950s, the first generation with a legitimate expectation of better treatment. They were perhaps also the first generation to have these expectations dashed.

We should also note the impact of the proportional growth of middle-class patients, suffering less serious problems, within UK psychiatry in the second half of the twentieth century (see Chapter 3). The middle classes not only bring more resources to a struggle, a fact which, combined with the less serious nature of their problems, increases the chances of them mounting a successful protest, they also tend to have higher expectations about how they should be treated, thus increasing the chances that their experiences of psychiatry will conflict with their expectations and generate strain. The middle classes expect more and are therefore more easily shocked and offended. To prove that this factor played any role in the formation of the MPU, I would have to demonstrate that the union recruited particularly heavily from amongst the middle classes, which I cannot do. Some of my interviewees, reflecting several generations of patient activists, bemoaned the overrepresentation of the middle classes amongst their own ranks (themselves included), but their claims are obviously impressionistic and, in most cases, do not refer to the MPU in any case. Nevertheless, the hypothesis is at least plausible and worthy of an airing.

*(ii) Structural conduciveness*   The reforms of the 1930s and 1950s are also significant in relation to the issue of structural conduciveness. They gave patients leverage for complaint. When psychiatry formed a part of the Poor Law and was expected to exert a controlling function, the claim that it was an institution of social control could carry little critical weight. That was the point of it. Similarly, during periods when 'lunatiks' have been judged less than human or equivalent to children they have had little basis upon which to make claims for civil rights. As the rationale of psychiatry shifted, however, from control to care, and as it sought to transform the image of those it cared for, removing stigma and insisting that they were everyday people suffering curable illnesses, patients acquired the rhetorical ammunition and social status they required to mount a critique. Psychiatry could be criticised for failing to live up to the image it presented to the outside world and/or on the basis of the standards which it claimed to establish. The environment was more conducive to protest.

Also important here is the effect of the move of patients from hospitals to the community, which had begun at this time, the increased use of out-patient services and the removal (following the 1930 Mental Treatment Bill) of the more custodial aspects of the mental hospital (see Chapter 3). An interesting way into this point is via Talcott Parsons' (1951) claim regarding the social control function of 'the sick role'. By means of this role, he argues:

> ...the two most dangerous potentialities, namely group formation and successful establishment for the claim to legitimacy, are avoided. The sick are tied up, not with other deviants to form a sub-culture of the sick, but each with a group of the non-sick, his personal circle and, above all, physicians... deprived of the possibility of forming a solidary collective
>
> (Parsons 1951, 477)

My analysis is rather different. Parsons assumes that the sick role serves to tie patients into relationships with doctors and their families, keeping them away from other patients with whom they might band together to form a group. The situation is not quite so straightforward in relation to psychiatry, however, since the old mental hospitals precisely brought patients into contact with one another, allowing networks to form between them. Like the churches and colleges that collectivised the black population in the south of the United States, facilitating the rise of the civil rights movements (McAdam 1982, Morris 1984), asylums collectivised mental patients. In addition, processes of diagnosis and 'treatment' assign a common identity to individuals who experience a potentially heterogeneous range of difficulties and put them in perceptibly 'structurally equivalent' positions within the mental health field. The psychiatric field thereby creates the very conditions for group formation and opposition that Parsons believes medicine undermines. The MPU was a union of 'mental patients' after all, and only those sharing the status and position of the mental patient were allowed full membership.

This is not to deny, as Parsons argues, that psychiatry was, for at least some of its history, largely capable of preventing collective action but, contra Parsons, this had less to do with the medical legitimacy of psychiatry or the sick role and much more to do with the sheer capacity for physical control embodied in the mental hospital. As 'total institutions' mental hospitals controlled the details of their inmates lives to a very intimate level (Goffman 1961). Even access to pens and paper could be restricted, making mobilisation very difficult. The asylum may, as Goffman notes, have had an underlife but this could not be converted into overt action. It was underground for very good reasons. Therefore the identities and networks created by the psychiatric system could not give rise to a movement for change. That is, not until regimes were relaxed and inmate facilities were joined by outpatient facilities, such as the PDH. I noted above, for example, that even in the 'enlightened' seventies, the formation of the MPU attracted harsh retribution in certain hospitals. Prior to the reforms of the mid-twentieth century, the conditions and controls were considerably harsher. In a system in transition between hospitals and the community, however, with a mix of hospitals, outpatient services and day hospitals, particularly progressive and liberal day hospitals such as the one at Paddington, we get a mix that is more conducive to struggle. We have a situation where patients are sufficiently networked to consider collective action but also sufficiently free of surveillance and control to be able to try. That the MPU began life at a progressive day hospital, which brought patients together without exerting 'total' control over them lends some support to this notion, as does the finding, cited above, that most members of the MPU were living outside the hospital. Many of these patients 'on the outside' would have spent some time in hospitals or day centres, such that they would be networked with other patients. Many, rejected by a wider society and stigmatised, may have lived their lives in what are sometimes seen as ghettoes of the mentally ill. But they were also free from hospital control and thus 'biographically available' for mobilisation, to borrow McAdams' (1988) term.

*(iii) Discursive formation and diffusion*   Even where structural conditions are conducive, however, strains do not automatically give rise to particular types of action. As the value-added model suggests, they must be interpreted or framed in a manner conducive to action. And if coordinated collective action is to follow, frames or the discourses which embody and embed them must be diffused through the relevant population. I noted earlier in this chapter that the two key discourses which framed *The Fish Manifesto*, anti-psychiatry and Marxism, soon became bones of contention within the MPU. This suggests that these frames did not resonate with a large section of the union's constituency. Neither discourse can be afforded too central a role in the process of mobilisation therefore. It might be truer to say that different frames mobilised different constituencies to attend the early MPU meetings and become involved, which is one reason why it was forced to federalise so early in its history. Nevertheless, it is clear that a hybrid composition of anti-psychiatry and Marxism provided the key framing for the early organisational committee of the MPU. Given the high profile and extensive diffusion of these two discourses in the sixties wave of contention this is a significant factor explaining the timing of the emergence of the MPU. Furthermore, in the case of anti-psychiatry at least, its critics within the MPU often owed more to it than they were inclined to admit. The discourse of the MPU was dialectically enveloped within that of anti-psychiatry, antithesis to its thesis. The fish manifesto is a clear example of this. It attacks anti-psychiatry but in anti-psychiatric terms. As such it pays homage to anti-psychiatry twice over; first, in the sense that it deems anti-psychiatry sufficiently significant to attack; second, in the sense that it borrows the language of anti-psychiatry. In addition, anti-psychiatry had exerted such a powerful shock within the mental health field that it is very difficult to discount its influence on the thinking of even those who seem quite independent of it. Anti-psychiatry had shaken up the doxa of the mental health field, allowing a range of different and competing views to

emerge. If these views did not always resemble it this is not because they were not influenced by it. The members of the MPU had to have a view on anti-psychiatry because of its centrality in the field of psychiatric contention.

As for the further frames/discourses which played a mobilising role, it seems reasonable, on the basis of MPU documents, to suppose that those of both civil rights and unionism played a part. Certainly both are prominent in these documents and it is reasonable to suppose, given their centrality in the politics of the early 1970s, that they would have resonated with many mental patients. Unions were important political players at this time. Any group with vulnerable interests and a claim to oppressed status might reasonably feel the need of one. Likewise, the heroic struggles of the black civil rights movement in the United States were still fresh in historical memory, even if they had given way to more violent tendencies by this point. Many groups were following the lead of black campaigners and claiming their civil rights, not just in the United States but throughout Europe. Civil rights discourse had become a 'master frame' (Snow and Benford 1992). It had permeated the language of common sense and it would therefore have seemed common sense to pursue one's interests under the rubric of civil rights.

*(iv) Trigger events*   In terms of trigger events it is clear, as noted earlier, that the strike at Paddington Day Hospital was central. The Paddington strike was where it all started. Without questioning that it was a key trigger event, however, it is important to note a few observations. First, the PDH strike was primarily about the PDH. It addressed the interests of workers as much as patients and did not, at least in any direct and immediate sense, threaten the interests of patients in other places. Second, as one might expect, considering this, the strike and events surrounding it only sufficed to mobilise patients from the PDH, and of these only one was recruited, after the strike, onto the original planning team for the MPU (the two patients who subsequently joined, prior to the first meeting, were not PDH patients). The strike did not have mass mobilising effect, therefore, and if we are looking for mass we might do better to look to such media events as the *Radio 4* interview. Third, and less unusually, the strike, or at least the events behind it, had to be framed in a particular way in order to serve as a trigger event. Smelser (1962) explains trigger events as very concrete events which symbolise wider and sometimes less tangible strains, giving them a concreteness and urgency more conducive to mobilisation. The psychotherapy sessions discussed earlier, which encouraged patients to think about the proposed closure of the PDH in terms of power and their own collusion, very much fits with this idea. The closure was framed so as to become symbolic of the very difficult situation that mental patients find themselves in. Nevertheless this symbolisation had to be worked at before it could be achieved. Like strain it had to be framed.

*(v) Mobilising structures*   In terms of the organisation and resources available for mobilization, two factors are particularly noteworthy. First, the

network of patients and sympathetic professionals generated by the movement of both between hospital units provided an important means for disseminating information about the inaugural meeting of the MPU. Channels of communication were in place. Furthermore, as noted, the very labels which were contested by the MPU provided the basis for a common identity amongst the constituent population. They were all 'mental patients' and could recognise themselves as such. In this respect the mental health field not only generated networks whose social capital might prove a force to contest it but more specifically what Tilly (1978) calls 'catnets', that is, networks whose members share a common category and therefore identity. Catnets are ripe for mobilisation in Tilly's view. Second, we have identified the role of agitators within and around the PDH, who played a key role in the early organisation of the MPU and whose previous experience in radical politics was an important asset – even if, in the final instance, their radical stance proved off-putting for some amongst the eventual constituency of the Union.

*(vi) Third parties*   The intervention of third parties, particularly the media and more particularly still *Radio 4*, played a central role in spreading the ideas of the movement and thereby boosting its recruitment. 'Mad lib' was a story with news value and journalists were keen to exploit the fact. Also important as third parties in this struggle, however, were mental health professionals. In the case of the MPU we can see these agents operating in two quite different ways. In the context of the PDH they effectively recruited patients into a strike and agitated in favour of the formation of a union. There is evidence, moreover, of other mental health professionals, in other settings, encouraging a supporting the union. However, we have also seen that some mental health professionals, in some settings, were very hostile to the idea of a union and sought by a variety of means to repress this development. The figures on involvement in the union, from both within and outside of hospital contexts, whilst they might be explained in a variety of ways, give us at least some reason to believe that this pattern was relatively widespread and was effective in quashing the formation of MPU cells in some places. Quite why some professionals would be positive about the idea of an MPU whilst others were negative is an issue which goes beyond this book but it is noteworthy that those professionals in favour, that we know about, were politically active in other respects, such that their attitude to the politics of mental patients may have been an extension of their more general political outlook at the time.

## Concluding notes

In this chapter, I have offered an account and explanation of the emergence of the *Mental Patients' Union*, the first key SMO in the 'patients' (later 'survivors') movement. As in other cases, I have sought to use my value-added schema to bring particularistic details and contingencies into a generalisable framework. Interesting comparisons could be made between the emergence of the MPU and other SMOs of the time, specifically those discussed in Chapter 6. Like PNP, for example, the discourse of the MPU was very deeply indebted to that of anti-psychiatry but it was also much more critical and the MPU elected to take on anti-psychiatry in a way that PNP never did. This might invite comparison with the NSF, but of course the two SMOs disagreed with anti-psychiatry for very different reasons and, as noted, the MPU actually accepted a great deal more of anti-psychiatry than their critiques might suggest. A further comparison with NSF might be focused upon the significance of the emergence of community and out-patient facilities. For the MPU, I have suggested, this marked a key shift in conditions of structural conduciveness which allowed the SMO to take shape. For the NSF, by contrast, it was the cause of the strain whose reso-lution was their very *raison d'être*. The same processes, it would seem, can play different roles in relationship to the formation of different movements and SMOs.

What is also interesting about the MPU, however, is the extent to which they illustrate the position taking which radical SMOs are sometimes inclined to engage in, perhaps on account of their structural equivalence, and which necessitates that we approach our analysis of them via their field. The MPU were not only critical of psychiatry or indeed of its apologists, such as NSF. They were critical of both but they were also critical of other critical currents including anti-psychiatry and MIND, investing consider-able effort in making these critiques (regularly). This process of critique, I suggest, was integral to the process whereby they attempted to build their own identity within the field of contention. One need not reduce this process, cynically, to a form of 'branding'. The disagreements of the MPU with both MIND and the anti-psychiatrists were, assumedly, quite genuine. However, their position, built as it was by way of critique of others, was inseparable from those others. It was a dialectical product of the ideas circulating and engaging in the field. In Chapter 8 we will see what became of these ideas in the late 1970s and 1980s.

# 8 Networks, survivors and international connections

In this chapter, I trace the development of the UK field of contention through the 1980s. I begin by picking up the thread of my accounts of anti-psychiatry and the MPU. I trace the flow of the former through Italian democratic psychiatry and the *European Network for Alternatives to Psychiatry* (ENAP) into an SMO called the *British Network for Alternatives to Psychiatry* (BNAP). The trajectory from the MPU leads to BNAP too, or at least through BNAP, but moves via a splinter group from the MPU who changed name various times but were best known as the *Campaign Against Psychiatric Oppression* (CAPO). Having discussed these various groups and their interpenetration the chapter considers the two SMOs who came to represent 'patient power' in the late 80s and who transformed the patient movement into a survivor advocacy movement: *Survivors Speak Out* (SSO) and the *United Kingdom Advocacy Network* (UKAN).

I shift analytic focus slightly in this chapter. Where Chapters 5, 6 and 7 were focused upon the conditions which give rise to SMOs my emphasis in this chapter is upon the issue of how movements outlive their founding activists and SMOs, and also how and why they change. In addition I have given more attention to the internal generation of movement culture.

## Trieste and *Psichiatria Democratica*

The ground which Laing and his colleagues broke effectively generated a new ground of taken-for-granted assumptions which a whole generation of activists were able to stand and build upon. If Laing had challenged habits of thought regarding the psychiatry of his own era, challenging the obviousness of psychiatry's assumptions and even its value, he left new habits and assumptions in their place. He generated an institution of anti-psychiatry. And as Merleau-Ponty says, institutions are not merely a sediment of the past but equally 'the invitation to a sequel, the necessity of a future' (1988, 108–9). Laing *et al.* set a 'game' in motion which developed a life beyond them and was destined to outlive and outgrow them – to change. Such change was achieved, in part, by way of the internal dynamics of the game itself. It was also affected by input from other national contexts, however, and other national variants of anti-psychiatry. Though perhaps the first genuinely 'anti-psychiatric' movement, UK anti-psychiatry was only one amongst a series of similar developments in the 1960s. Psychiatrists in many countries became involved in protest and found support for radical challenges to psychiatry from amongst philosophers, social scientists, artists and leftist groups. The best known of these developments, from a social science perspective, are the French developments: the radicalisation of the Lacanian school, the activities of Guattari and his colleagues (later including Deleuze), and the writing and activism of Foucault, Donzelot and Castel (Turkle 1981, 1992). A more important development from our point of view, however, came from Italy, in the form of the democratic psychiatry network, *Psichiatria Democratica*. Franco Basaglia, the figurehead of *Psichiatria Democratica*, had visited Laing and *Kingsley Hall*. He was impressed and aimed to create something similar in Italy. *Psichiatria Democratica*'s own experiment operated on a larger scale, however. Exploiting both a peculiarity of the Italian constitution and a crisis in Italian politics (a political opportunity), they were successful in bringing about a law which facilitated the dismantling of the old asylums. And in several towns in northern Italy, most famously the town where Basaglia himself was located, Trieste, this is exactly what happened. The asylum doors were thrown open and a radical form of 'care in the community' was implemented (Donnelly 1992, Kotowicz 1997, Ramon 1988).

*Psichiatria Democratica* had a different philosophy to the Laingians. Laing's philosophical base was existential-phenomenology and, in particular, its more individualistic, Sartrean variant. Though Basaglia was strongly influenced by Husserl and phenomenology, *Psichiatria Democratica* was solidly rooted in a Marxist (Gramscian) model. Unlike Laing they did not question the existence of mental illness or the use of, for example, physical treatments. Nevertheless, they viewed mental illness as an effect of alienating social relations and they believed asylum psychiatry to be a further form of alienation. Therefore they aimed to integrate the 'mentally ill' with the wider population; giving them jobs, locating them in the community and in some cases turning the old asylums into cultural centres for the local community.

It would be a mistake to attribute too much influence to Laing's circle in the processes which shaped *Psichiatria Democratica*. The Italian experiment was not a 'spin off' of UK anti-psychiatry. But it would also be a mistake to fail to appreciate that there was an influence and, in addition, that Basaglia and his circle were influenced by some of the same factors which had influenced Laing and his. The 'social psychiatry' and 'therapeutic community' movements within UK psychiatry, which had enjoyed a relative success after both the First and Second World Wars (see Chapter 3), were influences on both, for example. The very different context into which these influences flowed, however, both in terms of the 'external' environment of the mental health and political fields and the internalised social–political culture of the protagonists, ensured that they were appropriated and developed in very different ways.

The impact of the Italian developments on radical mental health professionals around the world, including the United Kingdom, was considerable. Radicals who were politicised by British anti-psychiatry, only to become disillusioned with it, but who retained an underlying commitment to the critique and transformation of psychiatry, found new cause for hope in the Italian experiment. As one activist recalled,

> I came to Britain...I was quite convinced that Britain had community care in place in mental health. I also, as I said, I was involved with the Laingian thing in '67, '68 and '69. I went to visit Cooper, where he was working in Shenley. I went to talk to him. I went to some of the seminars in London...I used to go regularly to Kingsley Hall and to the other community...I was convinced that there was a lot more of community care, in fact actually happening here. It took me a couple of years to understand that, you know the anti-psychiatry bit was totally isolated and had no bearing for the system. So I started to look around and to think, you know, does it exist anywhere? I was in the States a couple of times during the '70s and in fact in '82 I went to spend a month in community mental health centres in San Francisco, to see what they were doing there. And I was quite sure at the end that, the States, whatever is happening in the States, is not the solution. And then I read an article in *The Guardian* on the Italian thing, and I started to think 'how do I get to know it a bit better.'...And I met Basaglia, who cordially invited me to come and visit. [but he died before a visit was possible]... So I went to see Franca Basaglia [his wife] and she put me in contact with people in Trieste. And the person from Florence put me in contact with the people from Gorizia and that area. And I then went to spend a month in Contonia,[1] which is near Vicenza. And at the end of the same year I went for a month to Trieste. So until about '86 I would go for about for two months a year to different places in Italy.
>
> (Interview 4, mental health professional and activist)

This particular biographical trajectory is unique but it manifests a pattern which is common amongst mental health activists of a particular generation; a pattern of switching affections from the Laingian to the Basaglian model. The limits of the Laingian model became apparent and its impetus began to wane but the hopes and critical disposition towards psychiatry that it had aroused were not thereby extinguished. Rather, they were reinvested in a new model. Basaglia inherited Laing's crown, triggering a flow of new critical frames and practices from the Italian to the UK context. British activists rethought their project as a consequence of making contact with the Italians. They incorporated aspects of the Italian approach into their own.

A number of key activists within MIND were also impressed by the reforms. They both identified Trieste as a model of effective community care, against which the (in their view) failing UK model could be positively compared, and sought to defend it against certain critics, who argued that levels of neglect were in fact higher in Italy. Trieste became a point of contention in the field of contention and MIND lined up with the new generation of anti-psychiatrists in an effort to support it.

Following *Psichiatria Democratica*'s legal success, Trieste, like *Kingsley Hall* before it, became a place of pilgrimage, as well as a model to be aspired to. International intellectual 'stars' of anti-psychiatry were often to be found there, as one regular visitor indicated:

> Oh, yes, yes…Felix Guattari, I really met him mainly in Trieste because when I was invited there he was amongst the people they also invited, and er, what's the other guy's name? French guy? He wrote *The Psychiatric Society*? Oh, Castel, Castel. Both he, I and Guattari were, from time to time, invited to similar meetings. That's where it tended to be, in Trieste.
>
> (Interview 1, psychiatrist and activist)

> Well again I met Cooper because *everybody went to Trieste.*
>
> (Interview 1, my emphasis)

> After the German police cracked down on the whole [SPK[2]] thing a good number of those people, some of them I met, and some of them are still nurses of course, in Trieste.
>
> (Interview 1)

And it wasn't just the 'stars' who flocked to Trieste. So too, on a grand scale, did everyday radical practitioners. Indeed, much of the success of Trieste as an experiment was due to its ready supply of volunteer workers, all of whom hoped to learn from its liberated forms of practice (Crossley 1999b).

The general significance of Trieste as a 'working utopia' within the field of psychiatric contention has been discussed elsewhere (ibid.). I do not want to repeat that analysis here. It must suffice to note two direct ways in which Trieste had an impact upon the UK field of contention. First, it became an important locus of various forms of pedagogic endeavour and cultural diffusion. Because the 'Italian experience' was identified as a model of good practice, many critical practitioners from the United Kingdom visited Italy in an effort to learn from it:

> I've been back to Trieste about four times and one of the things that I did was try and move people forward in Manchester and try and get people more interested in what was going on…I organised sort of, about three or four separate visits and [name] did too…We either drove or flew groups of users and mental health workers to Trieste to see what was going on there. Stay for a week, have a look at what was

possible and using that to stimulate people to think about how they might do things in their own context.

(Interview 4, mental health professional and activist)

The first, literally what we did for the first week of the new team was, we all went off to Trieste. So we were a new resettlement team, newly sort of enthused, went over to Trieste, spent an incredible week, you know having our minds blown about it, and came back with a sort of, a kind of, what had been an emotional reaction against the things that we had witnessed and experienced in the hospital institution with a much clearer, won't say clearer, but much more robust kind of ideological understanding of the process of deinstitutionalisation... There was an element of evangelising, you known evangelistic feeling.

(Interview 5, mental health professional and activist)

There was clearly more to this than education, at least in a cold, cognitive sense. As the reference to 'evangelism' suggests, Trieste excited psychiatric critics, fuelling their commitment and giving them a sense of possibility. Indeed, the former of the two interviewees cited above spoke of returning to Trieste for a 'top up', capturing nicely the way in which it energised his activism. Trieste was a model and aspiration but also a resource to be tapped into. For this reason, moreover, as the second of the two interviewees noted, resources had to be made available for Trieste visits.

...we were very intrigued by it and basically wanted to keep up the link and continue the set up. We actually set up a Trieste fund. I was thinking it out, and we got a little logo and we set up [name], which was, the purpose was to set up educational exchanges in effect.

(Interview 5)

Furthermore, approaching the flow of Italian ideas from the other direction, a major UK visit by key players from *Psichiatria Democratica* was arranged.

People knew absolutely nothing about Italy. There weren't even misconceptions at that time. There were just no ideas. So we thought 'what can we do about that?' And together with the Italians we thought maybe we could bring some of them over to show what, to talk about what they were doing. Also to come with videos, with photographs, and they had an exhibition....

(Interview 3)

I invited them, it must be, dates are dreadful in my mind, 1985 or something like that. She and I organised the visit, quite a big visit of Italian psychiatrists and psychologists to England to have a...they visited everywhere in London, Manchester and Sheffield...

(Interview 1)

The visit was well received. As one interviewee, already cited above, remembers,

> [We] actually had a visit in Manchester, which was very exciting for us because we, it kind of stimulated us to think. It felt right. It felt very much where we were at and we put a lot of effort into putting our own manifesto together and used that as a kind of discussion document with them.

(Interview 4)

Trieste exerted a 'magnetic pull' for psychiatric radicals and animated them. Because of this it was able to distribute its forms of practice widely throughout the globe, including the United Kingdom. It was both the hub of a vast international network and the source of the most exciting experiment of its time. The effect upon the field of contention was consequently quite considerable.

One interesting spin off from this, in the United Kingdom, was the launch, in 1986, of *Asylum: A Magazine for Democratic Psychiatry*. This journal derived from 'the Italian experience' in a double way. On the one hand, as its subtitle makes clear, it was founded as a vehicle for discussing and disseminating 'Italian' ideas on democratic psychiatry. It amplified the process of discursive diffusion emanating from Trieste. On the other hand, its launch was funded by a financial surplus remaining after the abovementioned educational visit of the Italian protagonists to the United Kingdom.

The launch of *Asylum* was a key development. At a time when other outlets for psychiatric critique were drying up it plugged a central gap, regenerating a critical public and thereby helping to reproduce a national network of activists. Activists were kept 'in the loop' by *Asylum*. The founders of *Asylum* included veterans of the Laingian days, activists from the BNAP, which is discussed later, activists who were involved in the setting up of SSO, also discussed later, and a number of patients and professionals from around the Sheffield area, where the journal was originally based.

The second reason why Trieste was important was because, as the hub of an emerging network of anti- and critical psychiatrists, it became a meeting place where sometimes very different discourses were brought into dialogue, generating new hybrid discourses as well as new alliances and networks. One good example of this is the international *Hearing Voices Network*, a network born in Manchester (UK) but emerging out of a meeting, in Trieste, of representatives of the UK survivor movement with Marius Romme, a Dutch psychiatrist who had discovered both that many more people 'hear voices' than are ever 'psychiatrised' for it and that for many people hearing voices is not the problem that it becomes for some. Combining this idea with the idea of 'user empowerment', derived from the UK survivor movement, the network which emerged out of this meeting began to develop new and innovative ways of 'living with voices', many of which involved survivors working independently of the psychiatric system, and all of which involved a direct challenge to the dominant models of theory and practice in psychiatry. This network began as a small group in Manchester in the early 1990s but very rapidly spread both throughout the United Kingdom and further through Europe.

## ENAP and BNAP

The *Hearing Voices Network* was by no means the only or the first group to emerge from meetings in Trieste. The circulation of ideas and practices within Europe, around Trieste's magnetic pole, soon gave rise to a formalised network of European psychiatrists and mental health workers who were very critical of psychiatry: the *European Network for Alternatives to Psychiatry* (ENAP), also sometimes called the *International Network for Alternatives to Psychiatry* (INAP). They had their formative meeting in Portugal in 1974, and subsequent meetings around Europe in most years following, up to the mid-1980s.[3] INAP was, to a large extent, a 'talking shop'. As one early participant, a psychiatrist who had been involved in one of Laing's later projects, had worked very closely with David Cooper (who was also involved in INAP) and was later involved in setting up *Asylum*, explains,

> ... they issued a kind of platform... It was a kind of rough platform of ideas about the whole sort of mental health field in a sense and how the individual sort of countries could work on some kind of struggle. You could say in terms of creating alternatives to psychiatry. And Italy I think was, seemed very much as being in the forefront of changes within the area, I think. I think the idea of the network was really to bring together people from all walks of life, in a sense, so there was a kind of mixture of people who had been on the receiving end of psychiatry and people working in the field.
>
> (Interview 6, psychiatrist and activist)

By the early 1980s, a small number of UK (anti)psychiatrists and mental health workers were attending INAP meetings. Many, to quote another participant, had 'heard about the network from the people in Italy first' (Interview 3). This growth in British participation at the European level had the consequence that, following an INAP meeting in Brussels in 1982, a decision was taken to form a UK branch: the *British Network for Alternatives to Psychiatry* (BNAP). Slight differences in first hand accounts of the formation of BNAP emerged in my research. There is some indication, however, that its formation was prompted, in part, by a view aired at the Brussels conference that the British were insufficiently involved:

> They very much felt that there was a lack of involvement in the European Network on the English side. And people were wanting to know what was going on, that sort of thing. So David [Cooper] asked me if I would be willing to act as a sort of contact person for the English side and I said 'yes'. When I got back myself and a few of my friends, we started what became a sort of British Network for Alternatives to Psychiatry.
>
> (Interview 6)

Having been drawn into INAP by certain of his remaining contacts from his 'Laingian days', this interviewee subsequently set about drawing upon some of his other contacts from those days to form the organisational core of BNAP. Old 'Laingian' sentiments were tapped, old beliefs appealed to and old networks reactivated, albeit to give life to an SMO whose formal position differed somewhat from that of Laingian anti-psychiatry. How much BNAP did, in fact, differ from the earlier Laingian networks and how much 'democratic psychiatry' was re-read back through the lens of British anti-psychiatry is difficult to assess precisely – elements of both are evident in the archive. What we should stress, however, is that whatever changes were occurring were underpinned by continuities both in networks and in the basic commitment that gave them shape and held them together. Agents who had been politically socialised and networked during the Laingian era were regrouping in response to the impact of the Italian approach, which many of them subsequently assimilated.

Like INAP, BNAP was a forum for debate, although some campaigning took place too.

> We had a couple of meetings. We decided to meet on a regular basis. We wanted, obviously, to change views and practices in psychiatry. We were quite convinced that it is very important to listen to what users had to say and to follow it. And we were also quite convinced that the medical model is not the best model for psychiatry, and is also responsible for a lot of the problems. So we decided to go for specific campaigns rather than a very general crusade. And obviously to try to recruit people as well. We then had a couple of study days, one, in particular, about ECT and major drugs. We used the [London School of Economics]...as a place, as a space, but we also used sometimes [local] MIND [offices], especially in Hammersmith and Fulham, because one of the members was on the management committee there...
>
> (Interview 3)

> [BNAP] became a sort of forum really. We had regular monthly Sunday meetings. It became a forum, again a kind of open forum. Anyone was included that had an interest in the mental health field. We put on a few study days, a couple of study days, one about the closing of the mental hospitals and one about psychiatric treatments and that sort of thing...
>
> (Interview 6)

Although its London base made BNAP relatively inaccessible to potential recruits and established activists from outside of the area, it proved capable of attracting new recruits, several of whom went on to become key figures in the field themselves, founding further important groups and projects. It nurtured future 'stars'; socialising and educating, passing on both the cultural legacy of anti-psychiatry and a commitment to change. Furthermore, it drew in other strands of (anti)psychiatric critique which were emerging in the UK context. Alongside the various mental health workers who were involved in INAP and were enthused by the Italian developments, for example, BNAP attracted a number of radical academics who, at the time, were producing the first English translations of Michel Foucault's work on power, in their journal *Ideology and Consciousness*, as well as translations of important critiques of psychiatry and the 'psy' professions by Castel, Donzelot and others. From a completely different angle, BNAP attracted the participation of several members of a group whose origins lay back in the MPU (see Chapter 7). This group, who changed name frequently but ultimately settled on the *Campaign Against Psychiatric Oppression* (CAPO) were central players at this time. It is necessary to briefly trace their emergence.

## From the MPU to CAPO

In the aftermath of the dissolution of the MPU, as discussed in Chapter 7, former members went in different directions – including, of course, inactivity. Some joined up with PNP, who was still flourishing in the mid-70s. More significant, however, at least in terms of the history of the patients' movement, was a splinter group involving the founder 'patient' of the MPU, Eric Irwin. Irwin was unhappy with the organisational practices of the MPU, which he found too 'bureaucratic'. He thus split to form a group he called *Community Organisation for Psychiatric Emergencies* (COPE), a radical group who published two magazines at different times (*COPEMAN* and *Heavy Daze*), who operated at least one 'crash pad' (using Irwin's links in the squatters movement) and who maintained a radically anti-psychiatric and anti-establishment agenda.

COPE underwent numerous name changes. They reversed their acronym to become EPOC, before changing again to PROMPT (*Protection for the Rights of Mental Patients in Treatment*),[4] and then finally, in 1985, to the CAPO. The reason for this final name change, from PROMPT to CAPO, is important.

As two different PROMPT/CAPO members explained,

> ...some of us who were in COPE and MPU got together in PROMPT...
> That continued until April '85 when it was decided that we no longer
> wished to have the words 'patient' and 'Treatment' in the title. At my

suggestion we decided to change it to the Campaign Against Psychiatric Oppression.

(Irwin in Van de Graaf *et al.* 1989, 4)

The name PROMPT stood for Promotion of the Rights of Mental Patients in Treatment. The word 'mental patients' was in inverted commas [metaphorically speaking. Inverted commas were not actually used]. And in 1985 we changed the name to CAPO, *Campaign Against Psychiatric Oppression.* Although the word mental patients wouldn't be used these days this was like early days really. It's taken until the mid 80's to get away from using that word. Like other oppressed groups in society we have been, y'know, struggling with terminology over the years, finding the right way to describe things.

(Interview 7, survivor activist)

Although the medical model of madness, with its concept of 'mental illness', and the position of mental patients in society had been criticised by early activists, the term 'mental patient' had been freely and openly used between the 1960s and early 1980s. The MPU was a 'mental patients' union, for example, and PROMPT sought to protect the rights of 'mental patients'. By the mid-1980s, however, the oppositional culture in the field of psychiatric contention had begun to evolve. A new language, new labels and narrative forms were emerging, and the old language of critique was itself increasingly subject to critique (see also Crossley 2004, Crossley and Crossley 2001). The motor force behind this evolution was internal debate within the field of contention and the 'collective effervescence' it generated. New groups, such as BNAP, were forming, bringing new generations of activists into the field. In itself this brought new, more modern ingredients into the mix. In addition, however, debate and interaction were themselves a source of cultural (re)generation. Ideas were 'bouncing off' one another, giving rise to new ideas, new forms of self-identification and a new culture that most parties to the debate identified with but none could claim, individually, to have invented or coined. PROMPT members were important inter-actors in this network and the organisation itself, with its various manifestos and fora, played an important role. Indeed the PROMPT journal was the main anti-psychiatric newsletter in the United Kingdom in the first half of the 1980s. But PROMPT were overtaken by the very processes of cultural generation that they were contributing to and they found themselves out of step with the new emerging norms of what was becoming the 'survivor' movement. Radicalised 'mental patients' no longer called themselves 'mental patients'. New forms of self-identification were kicking in. Thus PROMPT became CAPO.

The notion of a process of cultural generation is integral to the concept of fields of contention. I want to further specify it in three respects. First, note that it is interaction which is culturally generative. I am not reducing cultural creativity to the individual. Clearly interaction presupposes individuals and their properties but it is, in itself, an emergent order and I am locating cultural generation at this emergent level. It is the process of interaction, the 'bouncing' of ideas, critique and counter-critique, which generates new practices and discourses. Second, social/symbolic interaction is an irreducible and non-linear system; each party affects and is affected by the others, and the actions of each only make sense in the context of the whole. As such cultural generation does not admit of simplistic causal analyses. Processes of cultural generation might be negatively constrained by aspects of their environment and inter-actors clearly bring a 'baggage' of pre-conceptions and sedimented experiences with them but the positive generativity of interaction issues from its own, irreducible dynamic. Finally, the generative and diffusion-related capacities of interaction constitute a common discourse and culture within fields of contention, which their participants assimilate in different ways and to different degrees, as PROMPT did. Participants orient to a common set of norms, a common vocabulary and a shared context of meaning. The meaning of their actions is increasingly dependent upon the cultural structures of the field and their ability to orient to them.

PROMPT's concession to the new norms of self-identification in the field should not be read as an indication of a more general willingness to 'toe the line' on their part. On the contrary, although they welcomed activists from other groups to their events and participated in the events of those other groups, they advocated a radical, uncompromising position and were often highly critical of other groups. As a 'patients only' group, for example, they always maintained a critical stance towards other groups, such as BNAP, which included mental health professionals. Furthermore, they maintained a strongly Marxist position, rooting their critique of psychiatry in a broader critique of capitalism and refusing co-optation into the 'capitalist system' by, for example, applying for charitable status (as some groups did) or assuming an economically rational organisational form, which is a legal prerequisite of official charitable status. Their only fundraising efforts were benefit gigs. Finally, they frequently described themselves as anti-psychiatric and as belonging to the 'anti-psychiatry movement' and 'the anti-psychiatry league'.[5] In these respects they were the true realization of the group called for in the *Fish Manifesto* – which is not surprising given that Irwin was behind both – and they assumed a very strong identity as radicals.

Although I have been unable to discover any definitive records, the ones that are in the archives suggests that COPE, EPOC, PROMPT and CAPO were a small group of more or less the same people. Some members left, others joined but the bulk of the members remained the same and that bulk did not at anytime exceed 20 members – though more people participated in certain of their activities and contributed to and read their magazine. This prevented CAPO from ever engaging in the mass protests that their references to 'class struggle' evoked but it effectively allowed them to avoid the problems of mass membership that had afflicted the MPU. And there can be little doubt that they made their presence felt in the field. Moreover, like BNAP they proved to be an effective recruitment filter, drawing people in to mental health politics who would later assume central roles. At least three of the key activists I interviewed had become involved in mental health politics via PROMPT/CAPO, for example:

> I first heard about the user movement... in about 1983. I read Judi Chamberlin's[6] book... At about the same time I heard of a newsletter called PROMPT put out by some survivors in London and sent for some copies. This was the first time I had known anyone else found ECT barbaric.
>
> (Interview 8, survivor activist)

This interviewee subscribed to the journal and began to follow the debates but, for both geographical reasons and a sense of unease at the sometimes aggressive tone of the newsletter, didn't become more actively involved until other groups began to emerge. The other two did get more involved, immediately:

> ... that was how I basically got involved, through CAPO. I mean I used to go to CAPO meetings. I never actually joined CAPO because in those days you had to kind of agree to the manifesto and I didn't agree with the manifesto [...] In retrospect, although I went to the meetings I didn't wholeheartedly support that...
>
> (Interview 9, survivor activist)

> It was in 1980. Before then I'd had experience of psychiatric hospitals, the psychiatric system and whatever, but in 1980 I came across a booklet produced by a group called PROMPT. Found it in a bookshop somewhere and a book by a group called, by Manchester Mental Patients Union. The book is called 'Know Your Rights in Mental Hospitals'. A group called the Manchester Mental Patients Union. I don't know if it still exists but it was around then. PROMPT was a London based group. But I found it all quite interesting and it was good to see that people are writing about the issues. And it was in August 1980 PROMPT were running a conference at Conway Hall and I saw a poster for it and I went along and I got, eventually I got involved in the group. And we did a lot of campaigning work on the streets.
>
> (Interview 7, survivor activist)

The three activists quoted above, to reiterate, were each to become central players in the field of psychiatric contention in the mid-1980s. That PROMPT/CAPO were an early point of contact for patient activism for each of them is therefore revealing of the importance of the group. Even if these would-be activists did not fully accept the PROMPT/CAPO 'line' (one did) they were nevertheless drawn into activism by the group. It was an important recruitment filter. The existence of a high profile group who were critical of psychiatry and trying to do something about it offered encouragement to those who had their own doubts about the practices of psychiatry, whilst the publications served as a gateway through to a wider anti-psychiatric literature.

CAPO became inactive in 1987, when Irwin died, and though attempts to re-launch it were made they did not, to my knowledge, succeed. The group was dependent upon his charismatic leadership and lost its basis with him. Nevertheless, PROMPT/CAPO were at a high point of their activism in the early 1980s, not least in their capacity as agitators and critics at BNAP events, to which I now return.

## Back to BNAP

BNAP were a loose network but also a point of centralisation within the field of psychiatric contention. Many of those who regularly attended their meetings and took part in their activities were also involved in other projects and groups, including INAP, the *Asylum* magazine, CAPO, *Ideology and Consciousness* and later, SSO. Initially BNAP provided a comfortable home for this diverse grouping and proved to be an effective recruitment filter, drawing in new activists and passing the history and culture of anti-psychiatric politics on to them. Tensions soon began to emerge, however. Accounts of these tensions vary. From one side, that of certain newcomers, there was a perception that BNAP, like CAPO, was a hangover from the radicalism of the 1960s and 1970s: '... to be perfectly honest they were kind of like Laing hippies really. It felt like they were very much on the fringe and not doing anything very practical' (Interview 10, mental health professional and activist). Furthermore, there was a feeling amongst some that they were too 'academic' and that their debates were too laboured and long, with no obvious practical outcome.

> It was a group run by mental health professionals and academics and that ... Personally I felt it was just really a talking shop. They set out to do certain things but nothing really came alive. . . . It did sort of seem to us that people didn't actually do that much. It's like . . . and turn it into like a talking shop.
>
> (Interview 7, survivor activist)

The academic disposition towards debate and discourse was not shared by the less academic or more practical participants and this resulted in a clash. Perhaps more important still, however, was a tension which developed between 'patients' (as they were still termed) and mental health professionals.

As one CAPO activist put it,

> The Network were heavily dominated by well meaning professionals. The survivors' input was very minimal.... There are issues that which are relevant like, that you weren't always encouraged to partake and through the nature of their job and profession some of these people will talk down to you and.... But there are other professionals who, in a way, maybe do come to listen but we should be sceptical of this.
>
> (Interview 7)

Some of the professionals welcomed the criticism that this generated.

> [BNAP] was a combination of professionals and users. There were sort of people from CAPO who came.... There was a guy called [name], who, he was quite critical of any mental health professionals involved in the anti-psychiatry movement. I always used to think 'quite right too'.
>
> (Interview 6)

However, the tension between survivors and professionals generated frustration for others. As one professional put it,

> ... it is very difficult, as I said, to get the users to be the initiators. There were always one or two or three people but not as a group. It was basically impossible to get them to work as organisers. To do a different thing. They would initiate a very good idea that, you know, that could potentially do a lot, but they were not at that time able to organise things. And I think that this was problematic because if the professionals were the organisers there was partly a sense of resentment, on both sides, of the sort of inequality, but also inevitably there was some imposition on say the structure of the day...
>
> (Interview 3)

This led to further problems: '...quite often decisions were not taken or were not followed up and, you know; organisationally it was not an effective organisation basically' (Interview 3).

These tensions were discussed in group meetings. Minutes for a meeting held on 23 February 1986, for example, record a discussion of the 'split between professionals and non-professionals in groups', further stating that,

> There was some feeling that the articulate members might talk down to others, but it was not accepted that the group would not be business like and caring. It was agreed that the issues raised were real and that easy solutions could not be expected. Further discussion was essential

and a number of alternative proposals were suggested [a special meeting was held to discuss these].

(minutes of BNAP meeting 23 February 1986)

What was happening here, I suggest, was that the structure and inequalities of the psychiatric field were being reproduced in the context of an SMO committed to challenging it. The professionals had deeply ingrained organisational dispositions. They were both skilled in organisation and inclined to take charge. This is what is picked up in the quotation from the survivor above who notes that 'by the nature of their job', some professionals 'talk down' to users. The survivors, by contrast, had been 'deskilled' organisationally by the paternalistic practices of the wider psychiatric field, as Goffman (1961) describes in relation to the asylum context. Their situation in the field was inclined to produce a disposition towards inactivity and dependency – though their involvement in the movement indicates that this is something they had elected to fight. This is what is picked up by the professional in the above quotations, who could not get survivors to do anything. Given that both parties were consciously committed to change, this inevitably generated tension, frustration and resentment on both sides.

Moreover the situation was exacerbated by the fact that many of the professionals retained a position in the mental health field and were committed to playing their political hand from that vantage point.

> ...probably we soften, the professionals, we soften the hard edge of the messages in the way we would convey it. I think either because we didn't want to burn our bridges or we wanted to make the message possible for professionals to hear, lots of issues around that.

(Interview 3)

On the positive side, professionals were able to use their 'feel' for the mental health game to devise ways of expressing criticism that other professionals would identify with and relate to. More negatively, however, the stakes were different for them and they had different inclinations. They had invested in psychiatry and therefore had more to lose by an outright condemnation of it.

The professional quoted above later reflected upon what she took to be a curious fact about the patient/professional divide as it was in the mid-1980s. Many of the professionals involved in BNAP, she argued, had themselves experienced some form of mental problem or had close relatives who had. And at least some of the 'survivors' had professional backgrounds and/or qualifications. Yet the division between the two camps was sharp. Everybody was forced towards one identity or another.

> ...there was all the time this insistence of making the distinction. So professionals were not allowed to be users and professionals. And at

the time there were very few people who defined themselves as users who also worked. There were issues about...labelling.

(Interview 3)

This insistence on maintaining the distinction persisted, moreover, in the group which succeeded BNAP, SSO. As the same professional reports,

> ...again there was no place to have a dual identity. But people like [name], who I met, I think, at the second meeting of Survivors, [...] She came to me at the end of the meeting and said, 'what a shame that the organisation cannot sustain the duality'. But it couldn't.... So, you know, professionals cannot vote, cannot be members of committees....

(Interview 3)

This is certainly an interesting development within the culture of the group. A rigid dichotomy was emerging between patients and professionals, and all participants were identified with one camp or the other, with no recognition of the many who fell into both categories.

This dichotomy, which played an important role in the downfall of the group, emerged, like the aforementioned rejection of the 'mental patient' label, out of a context of contingent interaction and debate. BNAP members could have looked at things differently and would have if the dialectical dynamic of their debates and interactions had moved in a different direction. However, it is important to acknowledge that there is a real basis to the distinction between 'professionals' and 'patients', even if professionals have been on the receiving end of psychiatry. Whatever their past experiences, as noted earlier, professionals have a stake in the mental health field, such that their attitude towards it will inevitably differ from that of the 'survivor' (whatever qualifications the survivor may have). With this point in view we can, I suggest, interpret the 'identity politics' that began to take shape within BNAP, between 'survivors' and 'professionals', as an effect of the very different interests and social positions of those groups as they are brought together in a single group.

## From BNAP to SSO

BNAP and CAPO, between themselves, were relatively successful in generating interest and concern in radical mental health politics amongst a new constituency, and in drawing already interested parties together. They generated networks and provided 'schooling' in oppositional dispositions and skills. They successfully cultivated a demand for change in psychiatry. As such they collectively constituted an important bridge between the first generation of anti-psychiatric radicals and an emerging new generation. Neither, however, was able to satisfy the demand which they created.

Moreover, both were, to a degree, overtaken by events in the field, in particular the formation of a new national 'survivor' SMO: SSO.

The crucial spark for the formation of SSO was a MIND conference in 1985, entitled '*From Patients to People*'. The aim of the conference was to foreground 'the consumer experience' and to this end 'consumer groups' (i.e. patient focused SMOs) and projects from around the world were invited to give presentations. Representatives of both CAPO and BNAP attended the conference but neither were invited to speak or present. CAPO thus opted for remedial DIY activity.

> ... there were survivors invited from Holland and America and some from Sweden as well, but no one from England. And we went down and set up a makeshift stand by the door just to cause embarrassment for MIND. The Dutch people were really nice people and they helped us to get a proper stall and got us in to some of the talks and gatherings which were going on during the conference .... 
>
> (Interview 7, CAPO activist)

CAPO's stall wasn't the only impromptu happening at the conference. The effect of the conference was twofold. First, the presentations by a variety of overseas networks and groups generated a shock recognition, for some delegates, of what was missing in the United Kingdom. As one founder member of SSO, who had previously been involved in both BNAP and CAPO, put it,

> What was noted by some of the radical workers there was that there was no movement, there was no; although there were individual survivors, well they wouldn't be called survivors then, but you know there were individual activists scattered around the country, there was nothing really going on in terms of co-ordinating action. And that was kind of pointed up by the fact that people from other countries, from survivor movements in other countries, from America, Holland in particular, but also Sweden were at that conference.
>
> (Interview 9, survivor activist)

In other countries survivors were organised in their own groups and they were beginning to make a splash. This inspired certain UK survivors to want to do the same. Second, the conference served to generate a national network which, in turn, formed the basis for a comparable UK development. Although the key discovery of the 1985 conference was the absence of a survivor network in the United Kingdom comparable to that in other countries, the conference allowed certain smaller-scale UK projects to come into contact with one another. Individuals and groups from Glasgow, Bristol, Chesterfield and London, amongst other places, connected and, following their own impromptu fringe meeting, elected to form a group. In the words of one of these founder members (who was involved in MIND, maintained postal contact with BNAP and was later involved in founding *Asylum*),

> ...we went to the National MIND conference. We took fairly radical steps. We actually went, myself, [name] and one or two other staff members. We went along with a busload of people using our services. We ran a workshop [...] this took a lot of people back at the MIND conference. It used to be a pretty staid affair. Certainly professionally dominated. And we received a lot of attention, a lot of positive feedback...making a very, a quite dramatic at that time, symbolic statement, you know [...] It was also there, at the 1985 conference, that a group of people approached us afterwards about setting up a network of Survivors and allies, which subsequently became known as *Survivors Speak Out*.
>
> (Interview 11, mental health professional and activist)

Following their initial, spontaneous meeting, the network's first step, as resource mobilisation approaches would predict, was to secure funds for a series of meetings. SSO was to be a national SMO, which meant that provision had to be made for potential participants from around the United Kingdom, who lacked their own funds, to travel to a series of meetings. In addition, those planning the meeting hoped to invite the Dutch users they had met at the MIND conference, to offer advice. A grant was secured from the King's Fund and the Dutch activists attended what became the first of a series of meetings (later SSO secured a further grant from the *King's Fund* and also a grant from MIND). A network began to take shape. As the above-cited founder member recalls,

> I committed myself to getting involved with that developing network, which subsequently involved me driving a bus down to the new forest to a place called Minstead Lodge on a series of weekends between 1985 and 1987, with people who were using our services. I'd take it from Chesterfield, pick up in Nottingham, and go down with me and about 25 other people for a weekend retreat and idea sharing and so on. It was user led but there were a couple of, a few workers, a handful of worker allies....
>
> (Interview 11)

It was during these meetings and the long discussions that they involved that the group, SSO, was formed and named. The process of naming was remembered by a number of participants as taking a long time:

> ...one of the weekends...was spent trying to identify a name. We started off with about twenty suggestions and we came down to *Survivors Speak Out*.
>
> (Interview 11)

... it wouldn't have been my decision. Other people would have had. I mean we used to spend hours and hours talking about things like that, y' know, quite rightly because it was, because that is how you get politicised, isn't it? But they were impossible debates. You could never get consensus. You can imagine.

(Interview 10)

Where the name actually came from is not clear. One of my interviewees noted that she was involved in the US co-counselling movement, who refer to themselves as 'mental health system survivors', and suggested that the name may have come from there. We should also note, however, that this was a time when 'survivors' of both AIDS and child abuse were beginning to achieve a public profile as self-identified 'survivors'. The survival frame was in circulation and had acquired an important symbolic value. In either case the naming of the group is evidence of both a transformation in the emergent culture of the field of contention and of a flow and movement of frames, identities and practices into the field from outside. And the consequence of this was that mobilised 'patients' began rewriting their identities. They were no longer 'patients' or 'mentally ill'. They were 'survivors' of both mental distress and the services provided to deal with such distress. The formulation of this identity involved a further break with medical discourse than had previously been achieved by activists and an attempt to 'take back' the right to self-identification. It also generated a new form of collective identification which linked survivors, past and present. Finally, as one early SSO flyer notes, it had strong positive connotations of which 'survivors' could be proud: 'The term survivor was chosen to portray a positive image of people in distress and people who experience differs from, or who dissent from, society's norms' (SSO, early information sheet).

The development of both this identity and the discourse in which it was nested was an important step in the development of survivor activism. Though it had antecedents, it marked the emergence of something new and different in the United Kingdom: the mental health survivor. As I have noted elsewhere, the survivor identity and discourse diffused widely and became commonplace (Crossley 2004, Crossley and Crossley 2001).

Money and discourse were not sufficient for the group, however. It needed members and a public profile, to which end it also needed publicity. SSO members therefore began contacting other potentially interested parties that they either knew or knew of: many local MIND branches were contacted, as were a surviving branch of PNP (with MPU links) in Manchester and a variety of London based groups and projects. In addition, SSO activists began to broadcast their emergence by way of articles and interviews in selected journals. Peter Campbell, the first secretary of the group and a key player in its early development (as well as later developments in *Survivor Poetry*) wrote a number of articles, for example, including one published in MIND's *Open Mind* journal, whilst Lorraine Bell, a clinical psychologist who played an equally pivotal role in the formation of the group, was interviewed in *Social Work Today* in a two-part article which also focused upon Dutch developments. These articles allowed SSO to give a clear indication of what they were about. Campbell, for example, discussed the group's first priority, to organise a conference for mental health consumers, and he emphasised that the group was not 'separatist', in the respect of being a 'survivor' only group, did not and could not represent all survivors, only those who engaged in its debates, and had no explicit manifesto or platform in any case. The point of the group was to allow 'survivors' to speak, whatever they may wish to say.

> Nevertheless there is a common feeling that the psychiatric system is an obstacle course to many who enter it; that the process disempowers; that psychiatry, ostensibly a series of enabling interventions, frequently disables; in short that psychiatry is something to be survived.
>
> (Campbell 1987, 7)

Bell echoed these points, adding that the network was not political; positively wanted to engage with professionals (and politicians), who had power and who might be persuaded to advocate for survivors; and wanted to constitute itself as a legitimate sounding board for future policy developments in mental health. Bell drew contrasts between the UK and Dutch movements when making these points, as the latter were both separatist and political, but the implicit contrast in what both she and Campbell wrote was with BNAP and CAPO. SSO were to be something different.

For their part CAPO and BNAP were equally suspicious. CAPO were critical of the role of professionals in SSO and both groups were unimpressed by the apolitical stance that SSO aspired to. BNAP minutes from 26 January 1986 document a discussion of Lorraine Bell's interview in *Social Work Today*, specifically noting, in scare quotes, the claim to be 'non political'. The minutes indicate that Bell had suggested that BNAP and SSO merge but BNAP was not interested.

Having said this, it is important to emphasise that SSO enjoyed overlapping memberships with both CAPO and BNAP, as CAPO and BNAP did with one another. This is represented in Figure 8.1, a network diagram based upon minutes of meetings for both BNAP and SSO, which also reveal the other affiliations of the members present (including 5 representatives with CAPO links). The overlaps between them facilitated a flow of information and ideas, enhancing the coordination and perhaps partly homogenising the groups. PROMPT's decision to drop the term 'mental patients' from their name and become CAPO, for example, reflects the linguistic politics

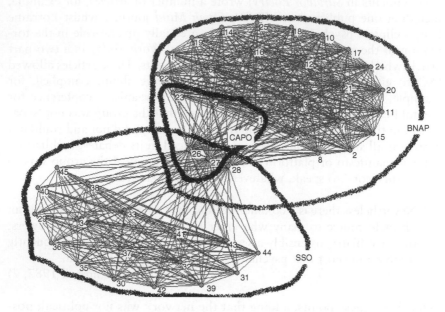

*Figure 8.1* Overlapping membership between BNAP, CAPO and SSO.

moving through this network. At the same time, however, the overlaps were a source of tension as they allowed contrasting viewpoints to clash. It is arguable that this weakened BNAP in particular, as its meetings were often the context where overlaps materialised. Both CAPO and SSO members attended BNAP meetings for a while, and both were critical (in different ways) of their host. Whatever the precise nature of the overlaps between the three groups, however, SSO was to be a project quite distinct from the other two and was to adopt a very different approach.

Early documents for SSO indicate that it began life as a coalition of a number of the pre-existing groups who had either met at the 1985 MIND conference or come into contact with the group subsequently. At an early stage, however, the network elected to function as an individual member-ship group, rather than an umbrella group. At the first count, in 1986, it had 20 members. After the early meetings, however, 'all of these amazing people starting piling in from everywhere' (Interview 11), and the group began to expand; rapidly at first, followed by a more gradual phase and then a further rapid rise. By 1995, membership figures had reached 565 (see Figure 8.2). The ratio of survivors to allies, at least between 1986 and 1991, was approximately 2:1. This growth in membership added to the legitimacy of the group, and improved its cash flow. Income from grants, such as those provided by MIND and the *King's Fund*, was

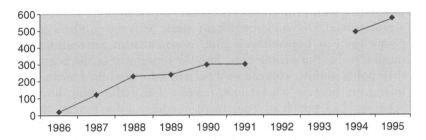

*Figure 8.2*   Survivor's speak out membership figures 1986–95.

Note
1992 and 1993 missing.

augmented by a yearly membership fee. With money the group was in a position to act.

The new influx of members, particularly members who wanted to become actively involved in the committees and internal politics of the group, also generated new problems, however. Or perhaps rather regenerated problems that, from the point of view of the broader history of the survivor movement, were somewhat older. The core organisers of the early SSO were a small, closely emotionally bonded group of both survivors and 'allies'; that is, sympathetic professionals and friends or relatives of survivors. As a small group they had been able to work together, pooling ideas and resources, and working together. As the group grew, however, and as many new survivors entered the group who were not on familiar terms with the allies, the status of the allies became a source of tension. Following an early AGM of the group it was decided that allies should not enjoy full membership of the group, and should not be allowed to vote on motions discussed at meetings. This led many of the allies and also some survivors who were angry at the way their friends and relatives were treated to withdraw from active involvement. One ally, who played a key role in setting up the group, explained to me:

> There was a kind of pretty healthy kind of working relationship between us which meant that we could, y'know, making majority decisions that not everyone felt completely comfortable with wasn't a problem. And then I think, after some years, obviously those close kind of personal relationships broke down because the movement became so much bigger, the membership became bigger. And it was unhealthy for a small cluster to be, y'know, hogging the show as it were. So, once the committee became voted in, there was new blood from different parts of the country, people that we didn't know so well, whose names I've forgotten because I didn't have such strong relationships with them but

some of whose names you'll know. People like [name]. So it, what happened then was, people like me, I wasn't a person. Like suddenly I was a professional. Do you know what I mean, 'Cos the numbers grew and people came in. I mean this is going to sound a bit patronising. I don't mean it to be. But people came into the movement at the beginning of their politicisation, whereas we'd been in it for a while. I mean it's very interesting because it's bit like, I mean that awful thing like people accusing black people of being racist to whites. I don't mean this at all. I'm not saying, in any way, my, the way people related to me had any meaningful parallel to the way other people are stereotyped at all. In terms of the kinds of implications of it there's no parallel whatsoever. But it became, let's say, less pleasant for me to be in the movement. And I'm not somebody who tolerates attack very easily. So that influenced, I think, my stepping down.

(Interview 10)

Part of what was going on here was the resurfacing of what has emerged in this study as an essential tension in radical mental health politics concerning the role of allies. At the same time, however, we can see the impact both of 'numbers' and of 'generations'. The growth of SSO meant that a whole new generation entered the group, a generation who had not been involved in its formation and who did not therefore share the culture and *esprit de corps* that had grown, organically, between the small core of founding members. They were inevitably going to challenge that culture and the cliquish bonds that invested it, and arguably had to do so if they were to take a part in the group, since these social formations excluded them. At the same time, as both Simmel (1950) and the earlier interviewee note, an increase in group size can necessitate a transformation of organisation, since some organisational forms which work very effectively for small group do not work as well for larger group. SSO had crossed a sociological threshold. Informal ties and rules of thumb, whilst ever present in any organisation, were no longer sufficient to hold the organisation together and gave way to formal mechanisms. Moreover, this 'rationalisation' brought to the surface potential tensions, between survivors and allies, that a more informal and personal mode of organisation had been able to work around.

## Culture

Before pushing on with the narrative, it is important to pause briefly to reflect in more detail upon the cultural shift in 'patient politics' that has already been referred to at a number of points in this chapter, a shift which requires me to refer now to 'survivor' rather than 'patient politics'. The emergence and rapid diffusion of a new discourse on mental difficulties, with a new vocabulary, imagery and rhetorical armoury, is very noticeable in the archive (see also Cresswell forthcoming, Crossley and Crossley 2001). In a short time, survivor discourse achieved dominance in radical mental health circles. Moreover, the discourse was attached to a specific 'repertoire of contention' (see Chapter 2). We can best bring this out by contrasting the groups of the 1980s with the MPU. The MPU were a 'union' who emerged out of a 'strike' and whose pioneers theorised their struggle as part of a wider class struggle. There is no such imagery in *Survivors Speak Out* or the related groups and networks of this time. Moreover, their techniques of protest are no longer approximations of labour techniques (e.g. strikes and demos) but rather consist in: the giving of testimony (see also Cresswell forthcoming); symbolic moments of silence for the victims of psychiatry; and the laying of wreaths. One activist, involved in the *All-Wales Network*, a prominent group in the mid-1990s, told me of the candlelight vigil his group had held outside a newly constructed ECT suite:

> ...they were going to build a new ECT suite attached to the local hospital and we campaigned pretty rigorously through the local press and candlelight vigils and things like that. Y'know, very touchy-feely direct action sort of things, based on a model that we had nicked from the disability movement...
>
> (Interview 12, survivor activist)

These changes may be explained, in part, by reference to the internal dynamics of the field. Fields of contention are always 'in process' and we should not be surprised if their elements change. Beyond that, however, there is also a clear resonance with HIV and child-abuse related forms of activism which were prominent at the time. And, in the case of the latter, one can trace a fairly direct line of influence via the early involvement in SSO of a constellation of Bristol-based women's groups, collectively operating under the umbrella of 'Bristol Women and Mental Health Network' (BWMHN). BWMHN activists were directly involved in the politics of abuse. It wasn't only 'patient politics' that had changed. The wider context of social movement politics in the United Kingdom had shifted. Industrial issues had dropped down the agenda and issues relating to the 'survival' of abuse and illness had risen up it. Furthermore, this shift had been accompanied by a shift in the repertoire of contention. Techniques of direct confrontation were now less often used and techniques of symbolically confronting pain more often used, at least in some activist circles. Mental health activists were part of that process of change, contributing to and shaping it but also shaped by it. Like the MPU before them, they formulated their politics in and by means of a political culture which pre-existed them, 'bending' this cultural material to make it properly serve their ends but working with it all the same. In doing so, of course, they were no different to any other social movement.

## UKAN

SSO was not the only SMO to emerge out of MIND's 1985 conference. The presentations at that conference by the Dutch group were sufficiently impressive to inspire a local MIND group in Nottingham, using a grant from their local health authority, to set up their own patient's council. Again the Dutch were involved in consultation. Numerous other groups followed suit or at least attempted to do so, prompting the Nottingham group to hold a series of cross-group meetings, followed by a conference. The result of this, in turn, was the formation of an umbrella group, initially called the National Advocacy Network and then subsequently the *United Kingdom Advocacy Network* (UKAN).[7] The purpose of UKAN was and is to provide a means for a whole variety of local user/survivor groups to be set up (starter packs are provided by the network) and to communicate and swap ideas.

The emergence of UKAN, with the many local groups that it embraced under its umbrella, running alongside SSO, strengthened the overall survivor profile in the field and reinforced the message that survivors had a voice and wanted to be heard. In these respects, the two organisations were complementary and enjoyed a relationship of mutual enhancement. However, they were also structurally equivalent organisations, seeking out support from the same constituencies and money from the same funding bodies. Inevitably, if not drawn into direct competition they at least felt a pressure to identify and mark out differences between themselves, as one former member of SSO explained,

> ...you could see straight away it was going to create problems if you had two organisations doing similar things. OK their membership, their structure, their constitutions are all very different, but in a way they are doing very similar things [ ... ] I often felt that people are really trying to make up reasons for, as to why they are different, but in fact, y'know, SSO had an information project, UKAN had an information project [ ... ] They were competing with each other for finances, competing with each other for people. 'Are you a UKAN person or an SSO person?'
>
> (Interview 9, survivor activist)

This is a 'field effect' and an illustration of why we need to understand SMOs in the context of their field. On the surface SSO and UKAN were separate groups, and of course each was a separate centre of decision making and action. But each impacted upon the other by way of their common links to third parties and each was aware of the fact, such that, at a deeper level, they were closely intertwined and mutually affecting.

## The fate of CAPO and BNAP

As noted earlier, CAPO began to wane with the death of Eric Irwin. Articles and interviews with CAPO members, chiefly commemorating Irwin's death, were published in such journals as *Asylum* in the late 80s but there is little indication of any other activity by this point. CAPO was more or less passing away as SSO was emerging. BNAP, by contrast, survived the birth of SSO, but it seems to have folded around 1989. The last set of minutes for a BNAP meeting that I have seen were for early 1988, an emergency meeting which was to address the future of the network and particularly the question of whether it should continue. The minutes indicate a decision that it should, albeit in a scaled down form, but this was the final hour. The group folded shortly after. The emergency meeting had been prompted by an apparent lack of support for the network, indicated by a drop in attendance at their meetings, amongst other things. Minutes for a meeting on 31 January 1988, where the emergency meeting was called for, indicate a number of possible reasons for the decline, some quite practical and contingent, such as a change of venue for meetings. There is also a recognition, however, of 'general apathy regarding Network', which was believed to be 'in part due to the proliferation of mental health advocacy groups'. BNAP had never enjoyed a monopoly on mental health radicalism but other groups, particularly SSO and UKAN, were beginning to emerge at this point who both had a broader potential constituency than BNAP and effectively drew constituents away from it. The new groups intended no harm to BNAP. They did not share the BNAP agenda but they welcomed its presence. Their very presence in the field of contention generated a 'field effect', however, which impacted negatively upon BNAP. They were structurally equivalent with BNAP, at the very least in the respect that they were pursuing the same constituents. Their gains were therefore always potentially BNAP's losses. BNAP, seemingly, could not survive the impact.

## Concluding remarks

In this chapter I have traced the anti-psychiatric and 'patient movement' trajectories from the 1960s through the 1980s. I hope it is evident that many of the 1980s developments were prompted by a momentum within the field of contention itself, inherited from the earlier periods of activism. Four themes have emerged as central within this narrative. First, we have seen that tensions between professionals and survivors emerge and re-emerge at numerous points. I have suggested that these wider roles and the power and interests attached to them often confound attempts to work together in radical mental health politics. Second, we have seen how SMOs enjoy overlapping memberships, such that they have blurred boundaries. This generates familiarity and rapport between them. They may not sing from the same hymn sheet but each has access to the hymn sheet of the other and there is inevitably cross-fertilisation. At the same time, however, it generates conflict because different viewpoints are in a position to clash. Third, notwithstanding this, we have seen how interactions within the field of contention generate a culture, of sorts, which affects all the parties to the interaction. PROMPT's decision to drop the 'patient' label and become CAPO is the key example of this. Finally, we have seen how the growth of a field of contention or an SMO and its duration across time generate new dynamics and issues. Competing generations have different ideas; a growth in numbers within SMOs affects organisation; a growth in (structurally equivalent) SMOs generates competition and tension etc. In Chapter 9 we see where all this led.

# 9 Consolidation and backlash

There are four parts to the 'story' in this chapter. First, I will briefly discuss the birth of two organisations, Schizophrenia – A National Emergency (SANE) and the *Zito Trust*, who, like *National Schizophrenia Fellowship* (NSF), were (and still are) opposed to overly liberal and anti-psychiatry. Analytically, I am less concerned with the formation of these groups, more concerned with the way in which opposition to existing discourse in the field of contention enters into the constitution of their identity. This illustrates the relational nature of SMOs as elements within a field. They are defined and define themselves relatively to their others. This applies to all SMOs, to some extent, but is very noticeable in relation to SANE. In addition, I want to use my focus on SANE and the *Zito Trust* to explore the nature of interaction between SMOs in fields, and in particular to show that and how division along certain frontiers within a field can generate temporary alliances elsewhere, where previously there may have been conflict or competition. The notion that a 'third' can generate identity and solidarity between previously unconnected parties is hardly new (e.g. Sartre 1969, Simmel 1950). It is important, however, as a further example of a field effect. It demonstrates that relationships between any two SMOs cannot necessarily be reduced to those two parties but must rather be understood in terms of the total constellation of a field of relations.

The second part of the story focuses upon the way in which the survivor movement, in the 1990s, was threatened by 'progress' which it had helped to secure. As opportunities for 'user' involvement in service organisation grew, I argue, the radicalism of the movement was threatened. Talented and motivated 'survivors' had alternative and in some ways more rewarding options open to them than conventional protest. This phenomenon puts an interesting spin on the idea of structural conduciveness. Hitherto I have framed my discussion on conduciveness in terms of the capacity within the mental health system for control and repression. Here I am considering the capacity of the system to absorb dissenters by bringing them 'on board'. This may be a positive thing. It may indicate a system which is genuinely representative of those involved within it. It involves compromise, however, which some may be inclined to criticise.

The third part of my story focuses upon the first stirrings of a third wave of quite radical survivor activism, based around two new SMOs: *Mad Pride* and *Reclaim Bedlam*. These SMOs really lie beyond the historical scope of this study and I discuss them very briefly. They are interesting, however, not least because they manifest a whole new protest style to that of SSO, and, as they appear to be influenced, stylistically, by the current wave of anti-corporate activism, illustrate my broader thesis about the ways in which mental health activists have worked within the broader protest culture of their day. As the MPU embodied the industrial politics of the 1970s and SSO the 'survivor' politics of the 1980s, so too *Mad Pride* and *Reclaim Bedlam* draw from the 'repertoire of contention' (Chapter 2) that gave us 'guerrilla gardening', radical Wombles, carnivals against capitalism and a politics of 'raving'.

The fourth part of the story, again only very briefly treated, focuses upon the massive growth of the number of survivor SMOs within the field and the increasing tendency for specialisation (of various kinds) amongst them. In the case of the latter tendency I believe that, again, we have a field effect here, one documented by both Durkheim (1964) and Simmel (1950). The growth of numbers of individual SMOs in a field, all in potentially struc-turally equivalent and thus competitive relations, generates a pressure for the newer entries to seek out a more specialised niche. Furthermore, if there are already large and successful groups dealing with 'issues in general' this frees up newer groups to turn away from the 'big picture' and address more specialised issues and concerns.

## SANE and anti-anti-psychiatry

Between themselves, SSO and UKAN represented the backbone of the survivor movement within the field of psychiatric contention through the late 1980s and early 1990s. Both played a crucial and central role promot-ing the voice of users, stimulating protest and calling for change. However, they were not the only new groups to form at this time. Another contender was to enter the field of psychiatric contention in the mid 1980s, and it was to make quite a splash.

SANE began life in a similar way to the NSF, with whom it shared a general outlook and to which it was originally connected. Award-winning campaign journalist, Marjory Wallace, ran a series of articles in *The Times*, between December 1985 and March 1986,[1] with the name 'Schizophrenia – The Forgotten Illness'. As with the letter that kick-started the NSF, this generated a large response. *The Times* received thousands of letters, many seemingly in support of Wallace's position. Initially Wallace channelled this support into her own support for the NSF. After a short period, however, inspired by the response to her article, she elected to form her own organisation.

Like NSF, SANE were and are primarily focused upon the problems caused by the shift to community care, a shift which accelerated following Margaret Thatcher's election as prime minister in 1979 (see Chapter 3). Patients were being moved out of hospitals and many of those who previously would have been hospitalised now remained in the community, but the community facilities necessary to accommodate this shift in approach were not in place. Community care was under-funded and mentally ill people were finding themselves on the streets, in prison or thrown back on families and neighbours who lacked both the training and the resources necessary to help them. Moreover, living now beyond the reach of the psychiatric gaze, many patients were failing to take their medication, resulting in greater rates of relapse and associated problems, including a small number of high profile attacks on members of the public and a relatively high and increasing rate of self-harm and suicide.

Some of the issues raised by SANE overlapped with concerns expressed by both MIND and the survivor groups. Wallace initially positioned herself on the side of the families of sufferers and the community, however, in a way which constituted mental patients as a 'problem'. In addition, her presentation of issues assumed a dramatic tone, emphasising what she saw to be the dangers which unsupervised 'schizophrenics' posed. Lack of government funding for research in mental illness, public prejudice and the failures of Community Care were all key concerns for SANE but these concerns were buried by the headline-grabbing message that unsupervised schizophrenics are a danger to both themselves and others. In itself this would have been sufficient to prompt a response from groups such as MIND, SSO and CAPO. The situation was compounded, however, by Wallace's explicit and very vocal critique of anti-psychiatry and other radical and liberal strands in psychiatry, which she claimed were complicit in, if not responsible for the closing of mental hospitals. Wallace had her own personal connections to anti-psychiatry, having been married to (and divorced from) a psychiatrist who had been involved in Laingian circles. In spite or perhaps because of this, however, she had very little sympathy for anti-psychiatry:

> [Laing's] ideas became weapons to scapegoat the family and especially the mother. These ideas may have appealed to sufferers but in the hands of clumsy GPs and social workers, they threatened the whole basis of family support. Laing's theories broke and still break the hearts of thousands of mothers who not only have to watch the damage inflicted upon their son or daughter by the illness, but are told they *caused* it.
>
> There is no evidence to support Laing's views but it is amazing how many people are still seduced...
>
> (Wallace 1992, 12)

In a perhaps unintended parody of the anti-psychiatric language of scapegoats, double-binds and 'insane situations', she sought to show how anti-psychiatric discourses make parents into scapegoats for the problems caused by schizophrenia and generate a series of 'Catch 22s' (double binds) which are themselves crazy. Specifically, in one published address she describes what she calls 'the treatment catch', 'the doctor's catch', 'the legal catch', 'the parent's catch', the 'family catch' and the 'awareness catch', in each case specifying how the logic of the mental health system, and more specifically the system as informed by liberal, left-wing and anti-psychiatric ideas, works in a way that fails both schizophrenics and their families (Wallace 1992). She is not, she insists, opposing the wave of humane reforms that began transforming psychiatry from the early twentieth century (see Chapter 3). But she is concerned that this: '...marvellous enlightened movement...became mixed with politics and with left-wing groups and anti-psychiatry movements which swept the United States and Europe. The idea was that by treating everyone as *normal* they would somehow become *normal*' (Wallace 1992, 12). Indeed, she claims that these left wing ideas provided a useful smokescreen for welfare bureaucrats looking to save money by closing hospitals: 'These ideologies now diluted and muddled by other agendas led to a secret and cynical handshake between extreme left-wing idealists and the apparatchiks of health services eager to cut the costs of keeping large institutions open' (ibid.).

The 'pendulum' of rights, she argues, has swung too far. It needs to be swung back. Moreover, she claims that most patients agree with her. Their interests, she argues, are misrepresented by a small minority:

> A recent survey in a North London mental hospital showed that 60% of sufferers who had been either detained in hospital or given medication against their will, were grateful for what had been done for them, whereas only 10% subsequently felt embittered. Unfortunately, it is that 10%, the vociferous minority, who have [attempted to] speak for the rest.
>
> (Ibid., 11)

We need to recognise that schizophrenia is a biologically based illness, she argues, and to focus our efforts into the bio-chemical research which will ultimately discover both its causes and its cure. To this end, SANE engaged in a massive fundraising operation to found an international research centre, based in an Oxford hospital and connected to the university there. In these respects SANE did not merely represent a different perspective to the more liberal and anti-psychiatric groups, as was the case with the NSF. Opposition to anti-psychiatry and to liberalism in psychiatry were integral to its identity and its agenda. It was an anti-anti-psychiatry SMO, and although that was not all that it was, it was a very central and visible aspect. As such SANE were bound to make waves and provoke conflicts.

A key battle, illustrative of the conflicts which ensued, occurred in 1988 when SANE launched a poster campaign on railway, tube station and bus shelter billboards in London and the South East. Their poster showed the face of a young man framed with the words 'He thinks he's Jesus Christ. You think he's a killer. They think he's fine.' The 'They' referred to here were liberal psychiatrists and liberal/radical critics of psychiatry. And the implication of the poster, though London commuters could arguably have read it in different ways, is that 'They' are wrong. The poster is a critique of liberal psychiatrists who do not use their power to diagnose and treat, compulsorily if necessary, as extensively as they should. This would have been enough to provoke those who called for greater liberalism in psychiatry. In addition, however, the further implication of the poster, if 'they' are wrong, is that there is some truth to the view that 'He' is a killer and certainly that 'He' is not 'fine', since he thinks that he is Jesus Christ. The poster makes its point at the cost of demonising the 'mentally ill'. For this reason it provoked an enormous backlash within the survivor and radical/liberal camps. Amongst its critics were members of MIND, who, though they felt that Care in the Community had been poorly implemented, did not share what they took to be SANE's view, namely, that we should return to a hospital based system. The editorial to the February 1989 edition of *Open Mind* opened with a response to the SANE campaign:

> Are we teetering on the edge of a new authoritarian age of incarceration – particularly for people with serious mental health problems? Big city public transport travellers might be forgiven for coming to this conclusion. That is, of course, if they could understand at all what the prominently displayed SANE posters were getting at. If they half closed their eyes, what key words stood out? Killer. Voices. Lies. Nothing. Jesus. Madness. Their conclusion might well be that not only did 'those people' inhabit some completely different world but also that 'those people' pose a particularly awful menace, the true dimensions of which can only be alluded to in public.
>
> (*Open Mind* 37, 1989)

MIND, CAPO, SSO and various local groups each sent letters of complaint to both the Advertising Standards Authority and to British Rail. The former, it was reported in the next issue of *Open Mind*, accepted that the posters could cause offence to some but held that it was not misleading because some schizophrenics manifest 'behaviour of the kind depicted'. The latter, though unsure whether the poster breached their code of standards, removed all of the posters and agreed that no similar posters should be allowed in future. In addition to this and as part of a range of publicity-generating activities for 1989 'MIND week', MIND launched a counter-attack in the form of their own poster/leaflet campaign. MIND's posters used the same face as the SANE poster but different wording: 'They say

I should be shut away, They say they know what's good for me, I have no say, Stop the neglect – MIND'. MIND were responding very directly to SANE's initiatives. Their campaigning activity was being shaped by their hostility to SANE. In addition a publicity war was beginning. Each side wanted to influence the attitudes and behaviour of the public and to counter the harmful effects of the views of the other. Moreover, certain groups, including CAPO, who had taken to protesting outside of SANE headquarters, stepped up their protests. SANE became a focus of activity and concern for groups such as MIND, CAPO and SSO. Having set itself the task of undoing 'the harm' that more liberal groups had caused it effectively transformed the agenda of those groups by becoming an immediate threat to be dealt with. Resources and efforts which might otherwise have been directed at psychiatry were directed at SANE. In terms of resources, however, SANE, though a relatively small group, centred upon Wallace, was much richer, at least in terms of the crucial resource of social capital. Wallace was a very well connected player, particularly but not exclusively in terms of the mass media. As an award-winning campaign journalist, she had both the expertise and the connections to operate effectively within media circles. She lunched with other leading journalists and with editors, giving her a significant edge over her much less media savvy and poorly connected competitors. Furthermore, she was able to use her status, expertise and connections to secure further important connections. For example, she secured financial support from the Prince of Wales (who is SANE's patron), from the Sultan of Brunei and many other notables. Royal and other 'high society' fundraising events were regularly reported in the *Sane Talk* magazine through the course of the 1980s. It is only because of this very high powered and high profile fundraising activity that SANE was able to afford to establish its own research centre.

Not all groups opt for strategies of elite patronisation. One cannot imagine CAPO attempting to contact Prince Charles' 'people'. Furthermore, the effort that went into securing and sustaining this support was immense, as I learned when I interviewed Marjory Wallace. As an individual activist, she worked extremely hard to secure SANE the standing, both financial and symbolic, it soon came to enjoy. But the intention and the determination are not sufficient without the resources. To secure resources one often needs resources, a Catch 22 in itself, and very often these 'start up' resources are not available to groups which take shape outside of elite circles. MIND, arguably, had once had enjoyed this level of resourcing, and though it may have fallen out with the establishment at this point in time it was still in a similar position of strength. It could call upon the great and the good if it needed or wanted to. For most groups, however, this level of resourcing exceeded anything they could aspire to. Moreover, SANE's advantage consisted not only in the group's resources but also in Wallace's considerable know-how in relation to the media 'game'. This became particularly apparent to me in the course of a series of interviews with the now defunct

*Schizophrenia Media Agency*, a small SMO, related to the *Hearing Voices Network*, which had grown out of Manchester MIND. The group aimed to lobby and educate journalists in an effort to combat the often very negative representations of 'the mentally ill' which they draw upon and reproduce. In addition, they offered journalists a 'supply' of survivors to appear on television or in newspapers and offered those survivors training in both the deconstruction of media images and the communication skills necessary to get one's message across clearly. The difficulty that the group experienced in even getting a response from many journalists, let alone a sympathetic response, contrasted very sharply with Marjory Wallace's accounts of media dinners and meetings with editors (Interview 13). She didn't always get what she wanted and was aware of an 'Oh it's Marjory again' attitude in some quarters (Interview 13), but the contrast could not have been more stark. And the 'skills gap' between the two was no less marked. Even when they did get coverage, the SMA often had difficulty getting their message across because they lacked experience of the media game. As an illustration consider the following activist's account:

> I did a quite a good article for, I forget which magazine it was now. [name] I think or something like that. And this was a very good article but we hadn't discussed the headline and they called it 'Don't hate me because I'm a schizophrenic' and I thought 'oh that's just failed the point, missed the point completely. It's not a question of love or hate. It's just acceptance. So I was very disappointed in that I didn't realise they would use, I mean that's a sort of headline which is the very thing you are trying to avoid.
>
> (Interview 14, survivor activist)

Marjory Wallace, by contrast, knew every trick in the book. SMA were learning but she was well ahead of the game and could play and use journalists, readers and unsuspecting others in much the way that other journalists could play and use SMA. On a number of occasions in my interview with her she spoke of 'doing the usual journalist's thing of . . .' (Interview 13), going on to describe how she effectively secured whatever she wanted or needed to make her story. Insofar as the liberals and radicals chose to take Wallace on in the media arena, they took her on very much on her home territory.

The interaction between SANE and the various other groups comprising the field of psychiatric contention, as with the interaction between SSO and UKAN, and between SSO and BNAP, reveals an important aspect of the field itself. Again we find that SANE, MIND and the others were not isolated atoms, nor did their relations consist entirely in direct bonds. They were indirectly connected to one another by relations of structural equivalence. They were appealing to the same social groups (politicians, psychiatrists, the general public, the advertising standards authority) about the same issues (mental health issues), on behalf of either the same or at least connected groups (survivors/patients and their families). Moreover, notwithstanding SANE's more extensive funding pool, they were sometimes appealing to the same funding bodies, again in relation to the same kinds of issues. These common links inevitably allowed each to indirectly affect the other and, as such, effected the irreducible interaction that is constitutive of a social field. Moreover, this interaction is intensified as each, inevitably, becomes cognisant of the other and begins to take the other into account in strategic decision-making. One cannot understand the behaviour of any individual independently of the structure of interaction constitutive of the whole. The others enter into the identity, the agendas and campaigns of each organisation. The definition of the other enters into the definition of self. SANE's explicitly anti-anti-psychiatry stance is a good example of this. Opposition enters into the very heart of the self-definition of the organisation.

In this case the relationships we are dealing with are primarily conflictual but, as Simmel (1964) notes, relations of conflict are no less social for being conflictual and are no less socially generative, even productive. SANE and to a lesser extent the NSF, who were closely aligned to them at the time, polarised the field. They became a target for the other groups and, to a degree, targeted the other groups. The 'greater evil' that they represented, whilst it did not eliminate all tension between SSO, CAPO and MIND, at least pushed them into a temporary alliance and gave them a common enemy. Thus by becoming a common enemy and immediate threat for a number of SMOs who were ordinarily in conflict with one another, SANE generated a temporary unity and coalition between those SMOs. Moreover, it is my contention that each side in this polarised field better represented for the other side 'the problem' than 'psychiatry' itself. MIND, SSO and CAPO encapsulated the liberalism that SANE believed bedevilled psychiatry whilst, from the other side, SANE articulated the social control agenda that MIND *et al.* believed to be lurking beneath the surface of the mental health system. It was easier for these opposing SMOs to mobilise against one another than against the more abstract 'mental health system', partly because the system was abstract and thereby elusive but also because their own positions were clearer, uncompromising and in conflict. Each was an easy target for the other. In this respect, the two sides fed off one another. Campaigning energies that might have been more directly focused upon psychiatry were focused upon the other but the provocation of the other provided an impetus to mobilisation which the various more heterogeneous and diplomatic voices of official psychiatry would never provide.

However, relations of conflict did not prevent these opposing SMOs from influencing one another in the 'mimetic' respect described by DiMaggio and Powell (1983) (see Chapter 1). In particular it is noteworthy that MIND, SANE and the NSF had all developed 'user' sections or forums by the early 1990s; that is, sections of the organisation run for and usually by 'survivors' (or 'users', 'consumers' or 'patients'). The reasons for this development are complex. Independently of the pressure which the constellation of SMOs comprising the field exerted upon its constituent members, a shift in government thinking at this time was ushering in a model of the patient as 'consumer' (see Chapter 3), which was increasing the symbolic value of the patient and in some cases attaching money to their involvement. Neo-liberal politicians were waging their own war on the monopoly and pater-nalism of welfare professionals, for their own reasons, and this generated a pressure towards 'consumer involvement'. In addition, however, the survivor voice was in the ascendancy as a consequence of the success of the survivor movement and its main SMOs (SSO and UKAN) within the field. This was contributing to the generation of a context wherein the survivor voice added legitimacy to an organisation and became necessary for those who wished to secure legitimacy. It made good strategic sense to have users on board because they had symbolic value but beyond that common sense, the bedrock of taken-for-granted assumptions that elude reflection (including strategic reflection) whilst shaping it, was shifting. It was becoming 'obvi-ous' that survivors should be involved in mental health debate, as obvious as it had once been that they could never be involved in a serious capacity. Moreover, for SANE and NSF the presence of a large body of users endors-ing their perspective went a long way to proving their contention that radi-cal survivors were a minority who did not speak for all service users, and indeed for demonstrating that their sometimes paternalistic sounding poli-cies were not only in the best interests of patients but also 'in tune' with the way in which patients themselves felt. It is impossible to second guess the exact motives which led the various organisations to adopt a user wing, of course, and it is against the spirit of a field analysis, in any case, to seek to reduce events to a single line of influence. What is clear, however, is that dynamics in the field of contention, which are traceable in part to the rise of the survivor movement and in part to a government focus on consumers, had generated a situation in which the survivor had a new, higher value, such that it was becoming both common sense and strategically advantageous for SMOs to develop a user section. One need only return to the 1950s, that is, to Chapter 4, to see that this was a quite historically specific state of affairs.

The emerging symbolic value of the survivor belongs to the culture of the field of contention, discussed in Chapter 8, and illustrates another way in which fields cannot be reduced to their players qua isolated atoms. Like the connections and relations of structural equivalence which bind players together, the culture and values of a field are relational. They emerge out of interactions but also act back upon and transform inter-actors.

## The *Zito Trust*

The battles in the field of psychiatric contention between SANE and the NSF on one side, and MIND, SSO and CAPO on the other, were to some degree self-perpetuating. One party would provoke another, who would respond in kind and so on. Wider processes and events inevitably impinged too, however. Government policy initiatives are one example of this but perhaps more dramatic, in terms of the mobilisation of energies, were a number of infrequent but very high profile incidents in which an individual who was deemed mentally ill and was living in the community injured or killed a member of the general public. One very significant case was the manslaughter in 1992 of a tube passenger, Jonathan Zito, by a diagnosed schizophrenic, Christopher Clunis. The story was one of very few which confirms the worst fears of the popular conception of mental illness; a schizophrenic kills a complete stranger in an open public place, in broad daylight, without any apparent motive. The incident provoked considerable media coverage, both initially and then later when a government inquiry into the event was published. And on both occasions this, in turn, was a call to arms for the SMOs comprising the field. All wanted to ensure that the story was reported and interpreted 'appropriately'; to ensure that the right implications and conclusions were drawn. As the NSF put it in their annual report for 1993–94:

> NSF fought to get media coverage for the views of its members. We had some success. The front page of the London Evening Standard carried the words of Eve Thompson, NSF's chairperson, as did reports in *The Daily Mail*, *The Guardian* and *The Daily Telegraph*. NSF spokespeople appeared on a variety of news and current affair programmes on Channel Four, BBC1, IRN, Sky Television, Radio Four and numerous local radio stations.
>
> As a follow up to this coverage NSF also arranged a nine minute slot with channel four news featuring NSF staff and projects ...
>
> (NSF Annual Report 1993–94, 12)

The Clunis affair was also the catalyst for the birth of another group, however, the *Zito Trust* (ZT), formed by Jayne Zito, the wife of the man killed in the incident. Following the incident Jayne Zito launched a massive publicity campaign, which involved a range of public meetings, appearances at conferences and television. As an articulate, passionate and attractive young woman, in a tragic, fairytale-goes-wrong situation, she had considerable media appeal and achieved a great deal of coverage. As such, moreover, she was a figure which many of the more mainstream groups were inclined to either align themselves with, or at least to avoid seeming to disagree with. For a time at least the field was behaving under the sway of 'the Zito factor' and nobody could avoid that. They might not like the fact and might not agree with Jayne Zito's take on events but she enjoyed a very strong symbolic presence and value and nobody could afford to ignore that.

The perspective which Jayne Zito adopted, at least initially, was most closely aligned to the more critical views of MIND, with whom she initially worked. She argued that incidents such as the one involving her husband were a consequence of policy failings and did not, in her view, provide evidence of a strong link between mental illness and violence: 'Ultimately, Christopher Clunis had to kill my husband Jon before he could receive the attention he so desperately needed. Why did he have to do something so terrible before anyone took any notice of him?' (Zito 1994, 5).

Over time, however, the perspective of the *Zito Trust*, as an organisation, drafted more in the direction of SANE's viewpoint, particularly as Jayne Zito herself adopted a more backseat role and handed over to a paid, professional campaigner. The two organisations worked together on occasion and came to be viewed with the same disdain from the other side of the field.

## Growth, consolidation and rebellion in the nineties

If the late 1980s saw the rise of 'another side' to mental health debates, in the form of SANE and the *Zito Trust*, it was also, initially, a time of growth for the survivor movement and its two key SMOs, SSO and UKAN. Both flourished. SSO became a public limited company and both achieved charitable status. This allowed them to secure further funds, which allowed them to pursue more ambitious projects, such as the 'information project' which both, independently (and competitively) developed. Both were able to move into offices, which for SSO meant moving out of Peter Campbell's living room, and both were able to employ workers in various capacities. SSO pioneered a '*Crisis Card*' scheme, which allowed survivor's to specify, prior to any subsequent breakdown they might experience, an individual who could be contacted and would advocate for them at a time of need – a right they enjoyed by law but which was often not realised, partly because such arrangements were often difficult to establish in the heat of the moment. In addition, again closely mirroring one another, both organisations developed an 'advocacy pack'; that is, a pack advising interested individuals on how to set up their own local group; how to secure publicity, recognition and funds etc.

The demand was clearly there. In their annual report for 1997–98, for example, UKAN listed 232 affiliated groups from around the United Kingdom. Many of these groups were small, local advocacy and self-help groups. By no means all of the groups fitted this description, however. This was also a time when a diverse range of more focused and specialised groups began to emerge; groups focused upon quite specific 'symptoms', such as the *Hearing Voices Network* and the *National Self-Harm Network*; groups who focused their critique upon specific treatments, such as the anti-ECT groups, *ECT-Anonymous* and *Shock*; and groups specialising in specific types and areas of lobbying, such as the *Schizophrenia Media Agency*. Moreover, at about the time that SSO had been forming, there was a noticeable growth of groups addressing the interface of mental health politics and that of both race and gender.

The advocacy packs and other infrastructural support that SSO and UKAN were able to offer clearly played a part in stimulating this growth. They spread the word, spread the expertise and, in the case of UKAN, served as a central hub in a wheel-like network structure, drawing groups in and connecting them. Small local groups could 'plug in' to UKAN and, via the group's newsletter, mail shots and (later) website, they were then in a position to both learn of the activities of other groups, publicise their own and achieve recognition from like-minded SMOs. Small, otherwise isolated groups who might have wondered what the point of existing, qua group, was were given the incentive of belonging, as an autonomous cell, to a national network whose other cells would recognise them and with whom they formed a wider movement. In addition, key activists provided an inspiration to become involved, as one local activist explained to me:

> There are lots of users, people like Peter Campbell, and people in *Survivors* [*Speak Out*] that have been around for years doing campaigning work. It makes you think its more worthwhile to be like them than to be sat in a day centre drinking tea and smoking and doing not much.
>
> (Interview 15, survivor activist)

The growth and shaping of the field of contention in the 1990s cannot be reduced to the positive aid and example of SSO and UKAN alone, however. At least three other factors were important too. First, the abovementioned diversification of the field betrays a dynamic of specialisation akin to that described by both Durkheim (1964) and Simmel (1950). New agents entering the field, who, at another time, might have sought to develop a generally focused SMO found both that there was no need for such a group, as groups of that description already existed, and indeed perhaps that there was no room for another such group. They could not afford to compete with other more established SMOs who would beat them in the competition for resources and support. They were able, but also required, to seek out a more specialised niche. Second, the emergence and diffusion of the internet and worldwide-web provided a new space in which relatively small and isolated groups, or even individuals, could participate in a larger network, connecting with others. The number of groups and individual pages on the web, dealing with experiences and views of psychiatry is vast. Finally, as noted above, a shift in government thinking which redefined 'patients' as consumers had created an environment in which the voice of the user was sought out and enjoyed a degree of legitimacy. Where the pioneers of the *Mental Patients' Union* had risked reprisals by speaking out and therefore had considerable disincentives to do so, consumer involvement was increasingly expected and, to a degree, resourced and provided for. The environment was becoming more 'structurally conducive'.

This latter development had a downside too, however, or at least its impact wasn't necessarily an unqualified good in the view of all. Many of the activists I interviewed had been involved in consultation exercises of various kinds and at various levels and most were quite negative about the experience. The committees on which survivors were enlisted were perceived by many of them to be overly bureaucratic and unresponsive – sometimes in spite of the acknowledged good intentions of those involved. Moreover, survivor groups struggled with such issues as to how they would and could represent their constituencies. Meetings often focused upon the discussion of lengthy documents made available a short time before the meeting. Decisions about these documents were going to be made at the meeting but there was no time for the survivor representative to consult their constituency. The participatory democratic ethos common to social movements came into conflict with the representative democracy presupposed by official committees.

Beyond committees, the new, more conducive environment enabled some survivors, individually and in groups, to set themselves up as consultants, consulting for health authorities, other survivor groups and a variety of projects. Their experience of mental distress, its treatment and of both resistance and the construction of alternatives was now beginning to count as 'knowledge' or 'expertise' within the system they had once resisted. They had a marketable form of cultural capital which they were able to use to improve both mental health services and their own circumstances. For some this was far more important and effective, politically, than sitting in on somebody else's committee meeting. When people pay you for your advice, one of my interviewees argued, they are more inclined to listen to what you have to say:

> Being able to influence things is not about influencing people because you are on committees or on planning groups. Real influence is getting paid to do consultancies and getting paid big, getting paid proper money, good money, same as any other consultant in the country would get. Because if somebody pays £28,000 for a piece of work they ain't going to ignore it, whereas often users are pulled on to these planning committees where they just sit there as a member of the planning committee and are basically ignored.
>
> (Interview 16, survivor activist)

This interviewee, a self-described socialist who nevertheless conceded that Margaret Thatcher had inadvertently helped the survivor movement a great deal by breaking up medical monopolies and encouraging self-help and a consumer led approach, recognised that the shift towards consultation may, however, have a downside for the movement. Another interviewee, also a consultant, spelled this out in more detail. He knew of about fifty survivor-consultants at the time of our interview (1997). On one level, he argued, their emergence represented real progress. The survivor experience was finally being taken seriously. However, this very success undermined the movement:

> whereas in the old days, say before up until the last three or four years, there were limited opportunity, if you wanted to do something. There were limited opportunities and so working unpaid for SSO or UKAN seemed like something worthwhile doing. Now, if you are together enough and you know, confident enough, you can go off and earn money. And maybe to jet out to Holland or Germany or the USA. I mean I have been to places over the last 15 years I never would have got to if it hadn't been the fact that I am, I am quite involved in the survivor movement. So what I think it has done is, some people who I think are, potentially might be leaders, have been sucked off into, you know. You become a free lance worker and rather than working, you know, ten hours a week. Well the ideas of working ten hours a week sticking envelopes for SSO or for UKAN suddenly seems to be much less attractive option. So I think we are in a second phase.
>
> (Interview 9, survivor activist)

Expanded individual opportunities and the availability of other ways of changing the system drew some potential activists away from the activist route.

In the very year that I was interviewing this activist, however, a new generation of activists were emerging and a new wave of activism seemingly taking shape within the context of SSO and local (London) MIND groups. One crucial spark in this regeneration was a proposal by the Maudsley and Bethlem Royal NHS Trust to celebrate the 750th anniversary of the founding of the Bethlem hospital ('Bedlam'). This provoked anger within some sections of the survivor community, prompting both a 'Reclaim Bedlam Campaign' and the formation of a direct action network, also named *Reclaim Bedlam*. In an advertisement in the *Survivors Speak Out Newssheet* in May 1997, the campaigners explained their position:

> As a User Controlled Group, we find the whole idea of 'celebrating' the history of Mental Health offensive. How can you celebrate LOBOTOMY, LIFETIME INSTITUTIONALISATION – TAKING YOUR OWN LIFE – DEPRESSION – DRUG DEPENDENCY ECT's and so on? It's our history and we should mark the 750th anniversary with our voice.

The group's first protest, 'Raving in the Park', was a 'summer solstice carnival' or 'social action DIY day' in Bedlam Park. Participants were invited to 'bring food, sound systems, activities, friends, family and just enjoy'. The purpose of the day was to 'acknowledge our survival and to call for the abolition of psychiatry and the destruction of mental health institutions and the professional and commercial interests who benefit from them'. 'Raving in the Park', which was dampened by the rain but still attracted about fifty participants, was then followed up with a meeting at St Paul's Cathedral and one minute's silence 'for people who have died of distress or at the hands of the mental health system over 750 years'.

When I interviewed the key activist behind *Reclaim Bedlam*, Pete Shaughnessy, who was also a member of SSO and had connections in local MIND organisations, he explained that it would continue as a direct action network. There would be no group, no committees, no bureaucracy, because he was weary of such things. But there would be periodic actions. And there were, at least until 2002, when Shaughnessy took his own life following a period of depression. That his death prompted an obituary in *The Guardian* newspaper is a testimony to the impact of his relatively short-lived campaigning career, but *Reclaim Bedlam* was no more.

However, *Reclaim Bedlam* was not the only new network to emerge at this time. Shaughnessy was also involved in another group, *Mad Pride*, formed by other members of SSO, which was to outlive him. The idea for *Mad Pride* seemingly derived from the London Gay Pride march in 1997 and a call for suggestions for Mad Pride events in the September 1997 edition of the *Survivors Speak Out Newssheet*. The group's originators felt that 'mad people' should have their own pride festivals and should reclaim the experience of madness as something to be proud of. Mad Pride statements and publications call for a celebration of difference and madness. The group has organised pickets and protests. Its main emphasis, however, is upon the promotion of mad culture, particularly music. Madness, they argue, is 'the new rock 'n' roll'. A number of gigs and events, including one to commemorate the death of Pete Shaughnessy, have been organised, and an anthology of 'mad stories', that is, stories which explore the funny and subversive aspects of madness, has been published.

The editors of the *Mad Pride* anthology claim that their group is 'set to become the first great civil liberties movement of the new millenium' (Curtis *et al.* 2000, 7). As such, they cross the temporal threshold that marks the end of this book. They are the 'to be continued' part of the story. Their emergence and that of *Reclaim Bedlam* are important and deserve a brief discussion, however, because they belong to a new generation of protest. On one level this generation revisits certain themes of past generations. The anthology, for example, includes, as the only historical piece, the famous 'Fish Manifesto' of the former members of the *Mental Patients' Union*. In addition there is a notable return to issues of 'class struggle' in their rhetoric, issues which effectively disappeared for a decade between the 1980s and early 1990s. *Mad Pride* and *Reclaim Bedlam*, however, are not throwbacks to the early 1970s. Their engagement in class struggle reflects a wider involvement in the events and culture of the latest protest wave to have swept the United Kingdom, and societies worldwide: the global anti-corporate movement. It is difficult to resist the assumption that *Reclaim Bedlam* borrowed its name from the radical, anti-corporate network, *Reclaim the Streets* (RtS) for example. Shaughnessy certainly modelled his network upon the latter, spoke at their events and was in contact with the RtS connected direct action newssheet, *SchNEWS*, who created a commemorative website for him upon his death. Furthermore he had enjoyed some involvement with the infamous 'Donga Tribe', whose opposition to the construction of a by-pass at Twyford Down formed a crucial chapter in the history of UK eco-protest. In addition, the decision to reclaim derogatory terminiology, such as 'madness', 'loony' and 'raving', resonates with similar re-appropriations in gay and black politics. And the focus on 'carnival', music, raves, DIY and protest as fun all bear the stamp of the wider culture of protest that was developing in the United Kingdom, and elsewhere, in the late 1990s; the culture that Naomi Klein (2000) would write about in *No Logo*.

There is an interesting and important pattern here. The anti-psychiatrists and the *Mental Patients' Union* each emerged at opposite ends of the '1960s' protest wave and each clearly belonged to their end of that wave in terms of their style, tactics, aspirations and connections. The anti-psychiatrists belonged to the counter-cultural beginnings of the 1960s, with its focus upon personal journeys, LSD and experiments in living. Its members were intimately interwoven with this scene. The MPU formed at the more politicised, Marxist-influenced and confrontational end of the wave, the era of the *Angry Brigade, the Black Panthers, Baader-Meinhoff* and *the Weathermen*. And they reflected this. They were a 'union', born of a 'strike'. They located patient politics within a broader class struggle and viewed their politics as revolution. And they enjoyed links with both claimants' unions and the *International Socialists*.

*Survivors Speak Out*, by contrast, formed in the mid-1980s. Leftist politics were still prominent and the United Kingdom was recovering from a year-long strike which had pitted an icon of the old left, Arthur Scargill, the leader of the National Union of Mineworkers, against an icon of the new right, Margaret Thatcher. The left had effectively lost, however, and the radical political agenda had begun to open up. True to their claim that 'the personal is political', feminists began to explore questions of child abuse, focusing their political energies on the many issues it raised. Simultaneously, as the HIV virus achieved its deadly visibility, the gay community channelled their collective energy into attempts to comprehend and make sense of what had happened within their ranks. Moreover, this was a time when the therapy industry was on the rise. Independent bookshops, which had once stacked their shelves with Trotsky, now stacked them with personal narratives of troubled childhoods and the process of recovery, with self-help books and 'depth' psychology. Finally, within the academy, Marxism and its economistic analyses was falling out of fashion – no doubt partly because communist regimes throughout the world, at this time, were either falling or shifting ground rapidly. Language and subjectivity were now hailed as the key terrain of struggle. It is perhaps not surprising then that the approach of SSO was more tentative and pragmatic, with a focus upon listening and speaking, making testimony and putting one's experience into words. And they enjoyed formal links to other relevant groups of the time, particularly feminist groups.

A number of my interviewees who had come to activism during this era expressed a view that the stigmatisation surrounding 'mental illness' necessitated that the protestors present a very rational face to the outside world.

> People with mental health problems have to be very wary about taking a public stance on issues because it's much harder for us to command public sympathy and public support in the, say than perhaps people with physical disabilities can. Do you know what I mean? Because there are all pervasive notions about mental health problems that come through mass, you know tabloid portrayals about psycho-killers or whatever it is. So people have quite distorted views. So we can to be careful about issues we take on publicly.
>
> (Interview 12, survivor activist)

> The emphasis is upon peaceful demonstration. I think that's really, really important. The media would have a field day wouldn't they? I mean if you look at it as a sociological point of view, there's a load of miners could end up brawling in the streets, throwing things about, angry for very good reasons. And people say 'oh right, we'll support them'. But if a group of psychiatric patients or ex-one's did the same, 'lock 'em up, they're mad'. And yet you've got the same. It's nothing to do with illness. It's to do with human rights.
>
> (Interview 17, survivor activist)

At the time this seemed compelling to me. Activists were anticipating the negative responses that angry protests might elicit and were designing their protests so as to avoid giving the wrong impression. *Mad Pride* changed all of that, however. *Mad Pride* didn't want to hide or disown their madness and quite explicitly rejected the tendency amongst their predecessors to emphasise that they were 'the same' as everybody else 'underneath'. They were, they claimed, different, and proud of the fact. Moreover they were critical of what they perceived to be the timidity, self-pity and political incorporation of their predecessors. Against what they perceived to be the strong tendency of survivor poets, to write of 'long, echoing corridors', they claimed that madness is 'as much to do with sex, drugs and rock n' roll' (Curtis *et al.* 2000, 8). In part, we can interpret this as a backlash against the old order, a rebellion of a new generation of protestors against the old, similar to the revolt against 'Laing hippies' amongst the early SSO activists. Every generation struggles to make its mark in a field and secure its succession. The wider political and societal context is important too, however. As I have already noted, *Mad Pride* emerged at a time when a new protest wave and a new protest culture were taking off. And like its predecessors, it too reflected the broader protest context within which it emerged and to which its various members were connected.

## Concluding comments

In this chapter I focused upon a number of developments in the field of psychiatric contention in the late 1980s and the 1990s. In particular, I have noted how the liberal and anti-psychiatric SMOs in the field came under attack from SANE and the *Zito Trust*, and how this generated alliances between the former. By opposing these SMOs SANE pushed them together and created a collective identity for them. In addition I have considered that and how the survivor movement of the 1980s became both a victim of its own success, qua movement, and, for this reason, an object of critique in the more recent wave of mobilisation, centred in particular on *Mad Pride*.

Interactions between SMOs are central. I have suggested, for example that conflict between SANE on one side and MIND, SSO and CAPO on the other were central to the identity and development of each. Each developed under the influence of its interactions with the others. Likewise *Mad Pride*'s rejection of the culture of the 1980s survivor movement illustrates just how embedded in it they were. It is integral to what they are that they are not like their predecessors. This negative relation is key. There is a lot more going on in the field than the interactions between its key SMOs, however. SANE, for example, like NSF, were clearly responding to the effects of community care policy and to such events as the killing of Jonathan Zito. Moreover, the incorporation of some of the 1980s survivor activists was related to a change in government policy which facilitated it. And *Mad Pride*, like each generation of survivor activists identified in the study, were taking up the new protest culture evolving in the United Kingdom and elsewhere at the time of their birth. Each of these processes and developments entered into and interacted with the interaction between mental health activists and SMOs, shaping what I have called the field of psychiatric contention. Fields of contention, it transpires, are immensely complex social spaces.

# Notes

## Introduction: researching resistance

1 Grant reference R000222187.
2 I have departed from this system, naming names, on one or two (but only one or two) occasions. These were occasions where the identity of the interviewee would have been obvious and using an 'anonymous' number would have threatened the anonymity of the interviewee on other occasions. On these occasions I was careful to ensure that my interviewees were only cited making claims which are in the public domain and attached to their name therein, in any case. I believe that this is closer to the spirit of maintaining 'anonymity' than a blank usage of numbers, even in cases where authorship is obvious.

## 1 Social movements, SMOs and fields of contention

1 As I discuss further later in this chapter, Zald and McCarthy have a very individualistic and economistic model, which fails to recognise the importance of social networks and symbolic interactions.
2 Technically (in social network analysis) broadcast networks are networks which involve the simultaneous diffusion of information (or whatever) to a large number of people, rather than on a one-to-one (node-to-node) basis. Generally they are also less discriminating. Media channels, which 'broadcast' information are an obvious example. Of course, notwithstanding 'call in' programmes, media channels tend also to involve one-way dissemination, such that my talk of interaction, in this context, may seem strange. However, it is well established in media studies both that audiences discuss media reports between themselves and, in some cases, 'shout back' at the TV or radio, either in support or disagreement. In this sense it makes sense to speak of 'interaction', albeit a type of interaction which differs from unmediated personal interaction.
3 'Minimal' is Hindess' term. He believes that we avoid problems in social theory by defining agency in minimal terms. I think that this can lead to problems, if all agents are reduced to their lowest common denominator but this is not necessitated by Hindess' argument and his use of this notion, to establish organisational agency, is persuasive.
4 I am referring here to anti-road and (airport) runway protestors who have occupied underground tunnels or tree-houses on a potential development site in an effort to stop trees being felled, bulldozers moving in etc.

## 2 A value-added model of mobilisation

1 Value-oriented social movements disagree with the values of their society or some system therein and seek to change these values. Norm-oriented movements agree

with dominant social values but believe that those values are ill served by prevailing norms, and thus seek to change these norms: for example, they challenge equal opportunities laws because they feel that these laws do not adequately realise the value of equality of opportunity.

2 Those who argue that they may not always be necessary suggest that 'movement entrepreneurs' can effectively generate 'grievances' in the cause of mobilisation (see Zald and McCarthy 1994). To my mind this implies that grievances are still necessary, otherwise why bother manufacturing them at all? However, the point is that mobilisation occurs in advance of the clear identification of grievances, a problematic but not preposterous claim.

3 'Freedom Summer' was a project organised by black civil rights groups in the summer of 1964. It involved bringing a number of affluent (often white) students from major universities in the North, down to the South to help the black populations with voter registration and related issues. The students met with great hostility. Indeed, three were killed in the first few days of the project. The popular film *Mississippi Burning* was based around these murders.

## 3 Contextualising contention: a potted history of the mental health field

1 Apothecaries are best described as forerunners of contemporary pharmacists. They prepared and sold medicines.

## 4 Mental hygiene and early protests: 1930–60

1 This citation was found at http://www.jhsph.edu/Dept/MH/History/index.html
2 MIND, as I discuss later, is the name that the group adopted in the 1970s; strictly speaking, Morgan is guilty of anachronism here as the group were not called MIND at the time she is referring to.
3 The *Royal College of Psychiatrists* did not exist at this point in time.
4 Royal Commission on the Law Relating To Mental Illness and Mental Deficiency: Minutes of Evidence (two vols), London, HMSO. NAMH gave evidence on the twelfth and twenty-eigth days.

## 5 Anti-psychiatry and 'the Sixties'

1 The anti-university was one of number of alternative educational ventures developed in the context of the 1960s counter-culture in London. It aimed both to teach topics (e.g. philosophies) not admitted on conventional university curricula and to reach out to communities ordinarily excluded from higher education.
2 Aaron Esterson, Sid Briskin, Clancy Sigal, Joan Cunnold and Raymond Wilkinson.
3 *The Divided Self* was not an immediate success but it became the best known and probably the best respected of his works when he became better known as an author.
4 Psychiatry and psychoanalysis are two quite different professions in the United Kingdom and Laing is quite unusual in occupying both positions. I refer to his psychoanalysis in the way that I do because it is fairly evident that, from the start of his training, he resisted and resented orthodox psychoanalysis and its institutional embodiment/hierarchy. He wanted the status 'psychoanalyst', which would provide him with the authority to practice and write, and he was attracted to some of the ideas of object-relations psychoanalysis (chiefly Winnicott) but he

clearly regarded much psychoanalysis as nonsense and managed to rub a good many psychoanalysts up the wrong way, including his teachers at the Institute of Psycho-Analysis (two of who attempted to block his qualification). On the positive side, he found much of therapeutic value in existential-phenomenology, eastern philosophy and LSD.

5 Durkheim uses the concept of 'Collective effervescence' in two juxtaposed ways in his work. Collective effervescence, when centred upon established festivals and rituals, can serve the function of reaffirming the status quo. Equally, however, he uses the term to capture the innovation and transformation associated with periods of social change and invention, such as the enlightenment and reformation.

6 This intertextual 'citation' was identified for me by a postgraduate student, Luke Caley, in one of my 'Social Movements' seminars. It was then pinned down to song, album and date, all off the top of his head (but later verified), by my PhD student (and chief music guru) James Rhodes. Thanks to both of them.

## 6 Parents, people and a radical change of MIND

1 So named because its full name consisted of two words, both beginning with 'P' (I've not been able to track down these words, just the acronym and its meaning). I felt qualification was necessary here in case the '2' in superscript led readers in search of a non-existent footnote.

2 A number of books were published with the main title 'Dianetics', only one has the quoted sub-title: Hubbard, R. (1968) *Dianetics: The Modern Science of Mental Health*, Hubbard College of Scientology, East Grinstead.

3 They brought cases against many organisations from many domains.

4 Pressures of space unfortunately.

## 7 A union of mental patients

1 The article was originally published in *Heavy Daze*, the journal of an SMO called COPE, whom I discuss in Chapter 6.

2 Technically a broadcast network is a network formed through the simultaneous and usually relatively impersonal transmission of information (or something) from a single source to multiple other sources. The mass media can be defined in these terms but they also 'broadcast' in a more everyday sense too. Node-to-node transmission involves one agent or 'transmitter' transferring information (or whatever) to either one other agent or perhaps a handful of specified others.

3 The official argument might be that more incapacitating treatment occurs in hospital because incapacitated patients require observation and hospital care. It is a common criticism, however, that strong sedatives are used in hospitals as a way of preserving order on the ward and making life easier for staff.

## 8 Networks, survivors and international connections

1 I may have misheard this name as it was unclear on my tape recording of the interview and I could not subsequently find it on a map of Italy.

2 As noted in Chapter 5, the SPK were a radical German patients' group whom the authorities linked with the Red Army Faction and who were therefore outlawed in Germany.

3 The meetings may have continued into the late 1980s and early 1990s but I have only been able to establish, for sure, that they lasted into the mid-1980s.

4 Some documents say *Protection for the Rights of Mental Patients in Therapy*. It is possible that the group were known as this but the more authoritative documents

say 'Treatment'. In talk the group were also sometimes referred to as Promotion of... Seemingly the acronym was more important, as the name of the group, than the precise wording it stood for.

5 As far as I can tell there was no formally organised 'league' as such. But CAPO did have international links.

6 A much cited US survivor writer and activist.

7 I assume it is intentional that UKAN, when uttered out loud, is 'You Can' – that is, you can speak for yourself, set up a group etc.

## 9 Consolidation and backlash

1 *The Times* 1985, December 16, 18 and 20; 1986, January 20, 23, February 17, March 3.

# Bibliography

Abbott, A. (2001) *Time Matters*, Chicago, IL, University of Chicago Press.

Appleby, M. (1963) Lord Feversham: A Personal Tribute, *Mental Health* 22, 138–9.

Bachelard, G. (1970) *Le Rationalisme Appliqué*, Paris, Presses Universitaires de France.

Barnes, M. and Berke, J. (1973) *Mary Barnes: Two Accounts of a Journey Through Madness*, Harmondsworth, Penguin.

Barnett, M. (1973) *People Not Psychiatry*, London, George Allen and Unwin.

Baron, C. (1987) *Asylum to Anarchy*, London, Free Association Books.

Berger, P. and Luckmann, T. (1979) *The Social Construction of Reality*, Harmondsworth, Penguin.

Berke, J. (1969) *Counter-Culture; the Creation of an Alternative Society*, London, Fire Books.

Berke, J. (1977) *Butterfly Man*, London, Hutchinson.

Beveridge, A. (1991) Thomas Clouston and the Edinburgh School of Psychiatry, in Berrios, G. and Freeman, H. (eds) *150 Years of British Psychiatry, 1841–1991*, London, Gaskell, 351–8.

Blumer, H. (1969) Collective Behaviour, in McClung-Lee (ed.) *Principles of Sociology*, New York, Barnes and Noble, 65–120.

Blumer, H. (1986) *Symbolic Interactionism*, Berkeley, CA, University of California Press.

Bourdieu, P. (1984) *Distinction*, London, RKP.

Bourdieu, P. (1993) Some Properties of Fields, in Bourdieu, P. (ed.) *Sociology in Question*, London, Sage, 72–7.

Bradbury, M. (1989) *The History Man*, Harmondsworth, Penguin.

*British Medical Journal* (1928, December)

*British Medical Journal* (1929, January)

*British Medical Journal* (1930, March)

Burt, R. (1992) *Structural Holes*, Cambridge, MA, Harvard University Press.

Busfield, J. (1986) *Managing Madness*, London, Unwin Hyman.

Busfield, J. (1996) *Men, Women and Madness*, London, Macmillan.

Cameron, J.L., Laing, R.D. and McGhie, A. (1955) Patient and Nurse: Effects of Environmental Changes in the Care of Chronic Schizophrenics, *The Lancet* 31 December, 1384–6.

Campbell, P. (1987) Survivors Speak Out, *Open Mind* 26, 7.

Castel, R. (1988) *The Regulation of Madness*, Oxford, Polity.

Clare, A. (1992) *In the Psychiatrist's Chair*, London, Heinemann.

Clay, J. (1996) *R.D. Laing: A Divided Self*, London, Sceptre.

Clouston, T. (1906) *The Hygiene of Mind*, London, Methuen.

Cooper, D. (1967) *Psychiatry and Anti-Psychiatry*, London, Paladin.

Cooper, D. (ed.) (1968) *The Dialectics of Liberation*, Harmondsworth, Penguin.

Cooper, D. (1971) *The Death of the Family*, Harmondsworth, Penguin.

Cooper, D. (1978) *The Language of Madness*, London, Allen Lane.

Cresswell, M. (forthcoming) Psychiatric Survivors and Testimonies of Self-Harm, *Social Science and Medicine*.

Crossley, N. (1998a) R.D. Laing and British Anti-Psychiatry: A Socio-Historical Analysis, *Social Science and Medicine* 47(7), 877–89.

Crossley, N. (1998b) Transforming the Mental Health Field: The Early History of the National Association for Mental Health, *Sociology of Health and Illness* 20(4), 458–88.

Crossley, N. (1999a) Fish, Field, Habitus and Madness; On the First Wave Mental Health Users in Britain, *British Journal of Sociology* 50(4), 647–70.

Crossley, N. (1999b) Working Utopias and Social Movements: An Investigation using Case Study Materials from Radical Mental Health Movements in Britain, *Sociology* 33(4), 809–30.

Crossley, N. (2002a) *Making Sense of Social Movements* (Chapters 1–3), Buckingham, Open University Press.

Crossley, N. (2002b) Global Anti-Corporate Struggle: A Preliminary Analysis, *British Journal of Sociology* 53(4), 667–91.

Crossley, N. (2002c) Repertoires of Contention and Tactical Diversity in the UK Psychiatric Survivors Movement, *Social Movement Studies* 1(1), 47–71.

Crossley, N. (2002d) Mental Health, Resistance and Social Movements: The Collective–Confrontational Dimension, *Health Education Journal* 61(2), 138–52.

Crossley, N. (2003) From Reproduction to Transformation: Social Movement Fields and the Radical Habitus, *Theory, Culture and Society* 20(6), 43–68.

Crossley, N. (2004) Not Being Mentally Ill: Social Movements, System Survivors and the Oppositional Habitus, *Anthropology and Medicine* 11(2), 161–80.

Crossley, N. (2005) How Social Movements Move: From First to Second Wave Developments in the UK Field of Psychiatric Contention, *Social Movement Studies* 5(1), 21–48.

Crossley, N. (forthcoming) The Field of Psychiatric Contention in the UK, 1960–2000, *Social Science and Medicine*.

Crossley, M. and Crossley, N. (2001) Patient Voices, Social Movements and the Habitus: How Psychiatric Survivors Speak Out, *Social Science and Medicine* 52(10), 1477–89.

Curtis, T., Dellar, R., Leslie, E. and Watson, B. (2000) *Mad Pride: A Celebration of Mad Culture*, London, Chipmunka Publishing.

Davis, K. (1938) Mental Hygiene and the Class Structure, *Psychiatry* 1, 55–64.

Diani, M. and McAdam, D. (2003) *Social Movements and Networks*, Oxford, Oxford University Press.

Digby, A. (1985a) Moral Treatment at the Retreat 1796–1846, in Bynum, W. and Porter, R. (eds) *The Anatomy of Madness Vol. 2*, London, Routledge.

Digby, A. (1985b) *Madness, Morality and Medicine: A Study of the York Retreat*, Cambridge, Cambridge University Press.

DiMaggio, P. and Powell, R. (1983) The Iron Cage Revisited, *American Sociological Review* 48, 147–60.

Dobson, F. (1998) *Frank Dobson Outlines Third Way for Health* (Department of Health Press Release), London, Department of Health.

Donnelly, M. (1992) *The Politics of Mental Health in Italy*, London, Routledge.

Durkheim, E. (1915) *The Elementary Forms of Religious Life*, New York, Free Press.

Durkheim, E. (1964) *The Division of Labour*, New York, Free Press.

Durkheim, E. (1974) *Sociology and Philosophy*, New York, Free Press.

Durkin, L. (1971) *Hostels for the Mentally Disordered*, London, Fabian Society, Young Fabian Pamphlet 24.

Durkin, L. (1972) Patient Power – A Review of a Protest, *Social Work Today* 3(15), 13–15.

Durkin, L. and Douieb, B. (1975) The Mental Patients Union, *Community Work* 2, 177–91.

Eisinger, P. (1973) The Conditions of Protest in American Cities, *American Political Science Review* 67(1), 11–28.

Elias, N. (1979) *What is Sociology?* London, Hutchinson.

Elias, N. (1982) *The Civilising Process*, Oxford, Blackwell.

Feree, M. (1992) The Political Contest of Rationality, in Morros, A. and Mueller, C. (eds) *Frontiers in Social Movement Theory*, New Haven, CT, Yale University Press, 29–52.

Fernando, S. (1991) *Mental Health, Race and Culture*, London, Macmillan.

Feversham Committee (1939) *The Voluntary Mental Health Services*, London, HMSO.

Foster, J. (1971) *Enquiry into the Practice and Effects of Scientology*, London, HMSO.

Foucault, M. (1965) *Madness and Civilisation*, London, Tavistock.

Foucault, M. (1972) *The Archaeology of Knowledge*, London, Tavistock.

Foucault, M. (1984) *The History of Sexuality Vol. 1*, Harmondsworth, Penguin.

Foucault, M. (1987) *Mental Illness and Psychology*, Berkeley, CA, University of California Press.

Goffman, E. (1959) *The Presentation of Self in Everyday Life*, Harmondsworth, Penguin.

Goffman, E. (1961) *Asylums*, Harmondsworth, Penguin.

Goffman, E. (1971) The Insanity of Place, in *Relations in Public*, Harmondsworth, Penguin.

Goffman, E. (1974) *Frame Analysis*, Cambridge, MA, Harvard University Press.

Goodwin, S. (1993) *Community Care and the Future of Mental Health Services*, Ashgate, Avebury.

Gostin, L. (1975) *A Human Condition* (2 vols.), London, NAMH Publications.

Gough, I. (1979) *The Political Economy of the Welfare State*, London, Macmillan.

Gould, R. (1991) Multiple Networks and Mobilisation in the Paris Commune, 1871, *American Sociology Review* 56(6), 716–29.

Green, J. (1988) *Days in the Life*, London, Heinemann.

Hervey, N. (1986) Advocacy or Folly, The Alleged Lunatics Friend Society, 1845–63, *Medical History* 30, 254–75.

Hindess, B. (1998) *Choice, Rationality and Social Theory*, London, Unwin Hyman.

Hinshelwood, R. and Manning, N. (1979) *Therapeutic Communities*, London, RKP.

Hunter, R. and MacAlpine, I. (1961) John Thomas Percival (1803–1876), Patient and Reformer, *Medical History* 6, 391–5.

Hunter, R. and MacAlpine, I. (1963) *Three Hundred Years of Psychiatry*, London, Oxford University Press.

Husain, R. (1992) Cast Your Mind Back, *Open Mind* 56, 15.

Irwin, E. and Hutchins, M. (1975) A Piece of Our Mind, *Heavy Daze* 2 (no page numbers).

Jack (undated) People Not Psychiatry: An Interview with Jack of PNP, *Red Rat* (further publication details not available).

Jenkins, C. (1983) Resource Mobilisation Theory and the Study of Social Movements, *Annual Review of Sociology* 9, 527–53.

Jenkins, C. and Perrow, C. (1977) Insurgency of the Powerless Farm Workers Movements (1946–1972), *American Sociological Review* 42(2), 249–68.

Jones, K. (1965) Community Care and the Mental Health Services, *Mental Health* XXIV(2), 60–3.

Jones, K. (1972) *A History of the Mental Health Services*, London, RKP.

Jones, M. (1968) *Social Psychiatry in Practice: The Idea of a Therapeutic Community*, Harmondsworth, Penguin.

Kesey, K. (1962) *One Flew Over the Cuckoo's Nest*, London, Methuen and Co.

Kitschelt, H. (1986) Political Opportunity Structures and Political Protest, *British Journal of Political Science* 16(1), 57–85.

Klein, N. (2000) *No Logo*, London, HarperCollins.

Kotowicz, Z. (1997) *R.D. Laing and the Paths of Anti-Psychiatry*, London, Routledge.

Kuhn, T. (1970) *The Structure of Scientific Revolutions*, Chicago, IL, Chicago University Press.

Laing, A. (1997) *R.D. Laing: A Life*, London, Harper Collins.

Laing, R.D. (1949) Philosophy and Medicine, in *Surgo*, June, 15(3), 134–5.

Laing, R.D. (1950) Health and Society, in *Surgo*, Candlemas, 91–3.

Laing, R.D. (1953) An Instance of the Ganser Syndrome, *Journal of the Royal Army Medical Corps* 99(4), 169–72.

Laing, R.D. (1957) An Examination of Tillich's Theory of Anxiety and Neurosis, *British Journal of Medical Psychology* 30, 88–91.

Laing, R.D. (1960) *The Divided Self*, London, Tavistock.

Laing, R.D. (1961) *Self and Others*, London, Tavistock.

Laing, R.D. (1964a) Schizophrenia and the Family, *New Society* 16 April, 14–17.

Laing, R.D. (1964b) What is Schizophrenia?, *New Left Review* 28, 63–9.

Laing, R.D. (1965) *The Divided Self* (second edition), Harmondsworth, Penguin.

Laing, R.D. (1967) *The Politics of Experience* and *The Bird of Paradise*, Harmondsworth, Penguin.

Laing, R.D. (1971a) *Knots*, Harmondsworth, Penguin.

Laing, R.D. (1971b) *The Politics of the Family and Other Essays*, London, Tavistock.

Laing, R.D. (1985) *Wisdom, Madness and Folly: The Making of a Psychiatrist*, London, Macmillan.

Laing, R.D. and Cooper, D. (1964) *Reason and Violence: A Decade of Sartre's Philosophy*, London, Tavistock.

Laing, R.D. and Esterson, A. (1958) The Collusive Functioning of Pairing in Analytical Groups, *British Journal of Medical Psychology* 31, 117–23.

Laing, R.D. and Esterson, A. (1964) *Sanity, Madness and the Family*, London, Tavistock.

Laing, R.D., Phillipson, H. and Lee, R. (1966) *Interpersonal Perception*, London, Tavistock.

Lemert, E. (1951) *Social Pathology*, New York, McGraw-Hill.

Lemert, E. (1974) *Human Deviance, Social Problems and Social Control*, Englewood Cliffs, NJ, Prentice Hall.

Littlewood, R. and Lipsedge, M. (1989) *Aliens and Alienists*, London, Unwin Hyman.
McAdam, D. (1982) *Political Process and the Development of Black Insurgency*, Chicago, IL, University of Chicago Press.
McAdam, D. (1983) Tactical Innovation and the Pace of Insurgency, *American Sociological Review* 48, 735–54.
McAdam, D. (1988) *Freedom Summer*, New York, Oxford University Press.
McAdam, D. (1989) The Biographical Consequences of Activism, *American Sociological Review* 54, 744–60.
McAdam, D. (1994) Culture and Social Movements, in Laraña, E., Johnson, H. and Gusfield, J. (eds) *New Social Movements*, Philadelphia, PA, Temple University Press, 36–57.
McAdam, D. (1995) 'Initiator' and 'Spin-Off' Movements, in Traugott, M. (ed.) *Repertoires and Cycles of Collective Action*, London, Duke, 217–40.
McAdam, D. Tarrow, S. and Tilly, C. (2001) *The Dynamics of Contention*, Cambridge, Cambridge University Press.
MacAlpine, I. and Hunter, R. (1993) *George III and the Mad-Business*, London, Pimlico.
MacDonald, M. (1981a) Insanity and the Realities of History in Early Modern England, *Psychological Medicine* 11, 11–25.
MacDonald, M. (1981b) *Mystical Bedlam*, Cambridge, Cambridge University Press.
McI Johnson, D. and Dodds, N. (1957) *The Plea for the Silent*, London, Christopher Johnson.
Marcuse, H. (1986) *One Dimensional Man*, London, Arc.
Marcuse, H. (1987) *Eros and Civilisation*, London, Arc.
Martin, J. (2003) What is Field Theory? *American Journal of Sociology* 109, 1–49.
Mead, G. (1967) *Mind, Self and Society*, Chicago, IL, Chicago University Press.
Mechanic, D. (1969) *Mental Health and Social Policy*, Englewood Cliffs, NJ, Prentice Hall.
Melucci, A. (1989) *Nomads of the Present*, London, Radius.
Melucci, A. (1996) *Challenging Codes*, Cambridge, Cambridge University Press.
*Mental Health* (1947–67), published by The National Association for Mental Health.
Mental Patients' Union (1972) *The Need for a Mental Patients Union: Some Proposal*, London, self-published pamphlet.
Merleau-Ponty, M. (1962) *The Phenomenology of Perception*, London, Routledge.
Merleau-Ponty, M. (1965) *The Structure of Behaviour*, London, Methuen.
Merleau-Ponty, M. (1988) Institution in Personal and Public History, in Merleau-Ponty, M. (ed.) *In Praise of Philosophy & Themes for the Lectures at the College de France*, Evanston, IL, Northwestern University Press, 107–13.
Miller, P. (1986) Critiques of Psychiatry and Critical Sociologies of Madness, in Miller, P. and Rose, N. (ed.) *The Power of Psychiatry*, Cambridge, Polity, 12–43.
Miller, P. and Rose, N. (1986) *The Power of Psychiatry*, Cambridge, Polity.
Miller, P. and Rose, N. (1988) The Tavistock Programme: Governing Subjectivity and Social Life, *Sociology* 22, 171–92.
Mills, C.W. (1967) Situated Actions and Vocabularies of Motive, in Mill, C.W. (ed.) *Power, Politics and People*, London, Oxford University Press, 439–52.
MIND (2004) *Fifty Years of Caring*, London, MIND Publications.
Morgan, E. (1997) *Fifty Years of Caring*, London, MIND Publications.
Morris, A. (1984) *The Origins of the Civil Rights Movement*, New York, Free Press.

Mullan, B. (1995) *Mad To Be Normal: Conversations With R.D. Laing*, London, Free Associations.

Musgrove, F. (1964) *Youth and Social Order*, London, RKP.

Musgrove, F. (1974) *Ecstacy and Holiness*, London, Methuen and Co.

*Open Mind* (1989) Editorial, *Open Mind* 37, 2.

*Open Mind* (1990) The Rights Stuff, *Open Mind* 47, 12–13.

*Open Mind* (1991) Looking Back, *Open Mind* 50, 12–13.

Parliamentary Debates (1929–30), London, HMSO.

Parliamentary Debates (1953–54), London, HMSO.

Parliamentary Debates (1958–59), London, HMSO.

Parsons, T. (1951) *The Social System*, New York, Free Press.

PEP (1937a) *Report on the British Social Services*, London, published by Political and Economic Planning.

PEP (1937b) *Report on the British Health Services*, London, published by Political and Economic Planning.

PEP (1939) *Britain's Health*, Harmondsworth, Penguin.

Piven, F. and Cloward, R. (1979) *Poor People's Movements*, New York, Vintage.

Piven, F. and Cloward, R. (1992) Normalising Collective Protest, in Morris, A. and McClurg Mueller, C. (eds) *Frontiers in Social Movement Theory*, New Haven, CT, Yale University Press, 301–25.

Popper, K. (1957) Philosophy of Science, in Mace, C. (ed.) *British Philosophy in the Mid Century*, New York, Macmillan, 153–91.

Porter, R. (1982) *English Society in the Eighteenth Century*, Harmondsworth, Penguin.

Porter, R. (1987a) *Mind Forg'd Manacles*, Harmondsworth, Penguin.

Porter, R. (1987b) *A Social History of Madness*, London, Weidenfeld and Nicholson.

Porter, R. (2002) *Madness: A Brief History*, Oxford, Oxford University Press.

Prior, L. (1993) *The Social Organisation of Mental Illness*, London, Sage.

Putnam, R. (2000) *Bowling Alone*, New York, Touchstone.

Ramon, S. (1988) *Psychiatry in Transition*, London, Pluto.

Rogers, A. and Pilgrim, D. (2001) *Mental Health Policy in Britain*, Hampshire, Palgrave.

Rose, N. (1985) *The Psychological Complex*, London, RKP.

Rose, N. (1986) The Discipline of Mental Health, in Miller, P. and Rose, N. (eds) *The Power of Psychiatry*, Cambridge, Polity, 43–84.

Rose, N. (1989) *Governing the Soul*, London, Routledge.

Sainsbury Centre (1998) *Acute Problems*, published by the Sainsbury Centre.

Samson, C. (1995) The Fracturing of Medical Dominance in British Psychiatry? *Sociology of Health and Illness* 17, 245–68.

Sartre, J. P. (1969) *Being and Nothingness*, London, Routledge.

Sashidharan, S. (1986) Ideology and Politics in Transcultural Psychiatry, in Cox, J. (ed.) *Trascultural Psychiatry*, London, Croom Helm, 158–78.

Schatzman, M. (1969) Madness and Morals, in Berke, J. (ed.) *Counter-Culture*, London, Fire Books, 290–313.

Scheff, T. (1984) *Being Mentally Ill*, New York, Aldine de Gruyter.

Schutz, A. (1967) *The Phenomenology of the Social World*, Evanston, IL, Northwestern University Press.

Scott, J. (1991) *Social Network Analysis: A Handbook*, London, Sage.

Scull, A. (1984) *Decarceration*, Englewood Cliffs, NJ, Prentice Hall.

Scull, A. (1989) *Social Order/Mental Disorder*, London, Routledge.

Scull, A. (1993) *The Most Solitary of Afflictions* (A Revision of Museums of Madness), New Haven, CT, Yale University Press.

Sedgwick, P. (1982) *PsychoPolitics*, London, Pluto.

Showalter, E. (1987) *The Female Malady: Women, Madness and English Culture 1830–1980*, London, Virago.

Siegler, M., Osmond, H. and Mann, H. (1969) Laing's Model of Madness, *British Journal of Psychiatry* 115, 947–8.

Simmel, G. (1950) *The Sociology of George Simmel*, New York, Free Press.

Simmel, G. (1964) *Conflict and the Web of Group Affiliations*, New York, Free Press.

Skultans, V. (1979) *English Madness: Ideas on Insanity 1580–1890*, London, RKP.

Smelser, N. (1962) *Theory of Collective Behaviour*, London, RKP.

Snow, D. and Benford, R. (1992) Master Frames and Cycles of Protest, in Maurice, A. and McClurg Mueller, C. (eds) *Frontiers in Social Movement Theory*, New Haven, CT, Yale University Press, 133–55.

Snow, D., Rochford, E., Worden, S. and Benford, R. (1986) Frame Alignment Processes, Micromobilisation and Movement Participation, *American Sociological Review* 51(4), 464–81.

Snow, D., Zurcher, L. and Ekland-Olson, S. (1980) Social Networks and Social Movements, *American Sociological Review* 45(5), 787–801.

Snyder, D. and Tilly, C. (1972) Hardship and Collective Violence in France, 1830 to 1960, *American Sociological Review* 37, 520–32.

Spandler, H. (1992) To Make An Army Out Of Illness: The History of the Social Patients Collective, *Asylum* 6(4), 4–16.

Steinberg, M. (1995) The Roar of the Crowd, in Traugott, M. (ed.) *Repertoires and Cycles of Collective Action*, London, Duke, 57–88.

Steinberg, M. (1999) The Talk and Back Talk of Collective Action; A Dialogic Analysis of Repertoires of Discourse among Nineteenth-Century English Cotton Spinners, *American Journal of Sociology* 105(3), 736–80.

Stone, M. (1986) Shell Shock and the Psychologists, in Bynum, W. and Porter, R. (eds) *The Anatomy of Madness Vol. 2*, London, Routledge, 242–71.

Szasz, T. (1972) *The Myth of Mental Illness*, St Albans, Granada.

Tantam, D. (1991) The Anti-Psychiatry Movement, in Berrios, G. and Freeman, H. (eds) *150 Years of British Psychiatry 1841–1991*, London, Gaskell, 333–50.

Tarrow, S. (1995) Cycles of Collective Action, in Traugott, M. (ed.) *Repertoires and Cycles of Collective Action*, London, Duke University Press, 89–116.

Tarrow, S. (1998) *Power in Movement*, Cambridge, Cambridge University Press.

Thompson, E. (1993) *Customs in Common*, Harmondsworth, Penguin.

Thomson, M. (1995) Mental Hygiene as an International Movement, in Weindling, P. (ed.) *International Health Organisations and Movements 1918–1939*, Cambridge, Cambridge University Press.

Thomson, M. (1998) *The Problem of Mental Deficiency*, Oxford, Oxford University Press.

Tilly, C. (1977) Getting it Together in Burgundy, *Theory and Society* 4, 479–504.

Tilly, C. (1978) *From Mobilisation to Revolution*, Reading, MA, Addison Wesley.

Tilly, C. (1986) European Violence and Collective Violence since 1700, *Social Research* 53, 159–84.

Tilly, C. (1995) Contentious Repertoires in Great Britain, 1758–1834, in Traugott, M. (ed.) *Repertoires and Cycles of Collective Action*, London, Duke, 15–42.

Traugott, M. (ed.) (1995) *Repertoires and Cycles of Collective Action*, London, Duke.

Turkle, S. (1981) French Anti-Psychiatry, in Ingle, D. (ed.) *Critical Psychiatry: the Politics of Mental Health*, Harmondsworth, Penguin, 150–83.

Turkle, S. (1992) *Psychoanalytic Politics*, London, Free Association Books.

Ussher, J. (1991) *Women's Madness*, Brighton, Harvester.

Van der Graaf, H., Irwin, E. and Bangay, F. (1989) The CAPO Interview (in two parts) *Asylum: A Magazine for Democratic Psychiatry* 3(3), 4–8 and 4(1), 5–8.

Wallace, M. (1992) *Schizophrenia 1992: Catch 22*, London, SANE Pamphlet.

Wallis, R. (1973) Convert or Subvert, *The Spectator* (29 December).

Wallis, R. (1976) *The Road to Total Freedom: A Sociological Analysis of Scientology*, London, Heinemann.

Zald, M. and McCarthy, J. (1994) *Social Movements in an Organisational Society*, New Jersey, Transaction.

Zito, J. (1994) Interview, *Open Mind* 67, 5–7.

# Index